# Something's Wrong

# Something's Wrong

When Life Gives You Lyme—
What's Killing Me Could Be Killing You Too

LISA R. CHURCH

RESOURCE *Publications* • Eugene, Oregon

SOMETHING'S WRONG
When Life Gives You Lyme—What's Killing Me Could Be Killing You Too

Copyright © 2019 Lisa R. Church. All rights reserved. Except for brief quotations in critical publications or reviews, no part of this book may be reproduced in any manner without prior written permission from the publisher. Write: Permissions, Wipf and Stock Publishers, 199 W. 8th Ave., Suite 3, Eugene, OR 97401.

Resource Publications
An Imprint of Wipf and Stock Publishers
199 W. 8th Ave., Suite 3
Eugene, OR 97401

www.wipfandstock.com

PAPERBACK ISBN: 978-1-5326-9886-6
HARDCOVER ISBN: 978-1-5326-9887-3
EBOOK ISBN: 978-1-5326-9888-0

Manufactured in the U.S.A.  04/18/19

Dedicated to my family.
Without them, I would not have survived this crisis.

*The following story has been pieced together from my snippets of memories from the summer of 2012. My family and friends filled in the blanks as best they could. It is based on the truth, but not all instances may be accurate.*

# THE BEGINNING

"Hey, girl! What's up?

Rose's relaxed tone, on the other end of the line, usually calmed me down. Not today.

"I'm pregnant."

It was the first time I'd said the words out loud. Hearing them was a punch in the gut.

"You're kidding."

My friend's jesting response irritated me.

"I wish I was. God, I wish I was!" I could think of nothing worse.

"Lisa, are you sure?"

"Rose, I've had three kids. I know how it feels to be pregnant!"

My friend's response was hesitant and still rather light-hearted. "I know, but I thought you went through menopause? Honey, you're 51 years old. Women your age don't go through menopause, then a year later get pregnant!"

"I know, I know," I said, trying to convince myself. "But the signs are here. I'm so tired I can hardly function. I'm nauseous most of the time—just like I was with Callie. And my entire hormone level is making me crazy! Hot flashes, dizziness, everything's the same, Rose. I haven't felt this way in years!"

I could tell my friend was thrown. There were no words for what she must have been thinking. I found her silence frightening.

"How long has this been going on?"

This answer rolled off my tongue easily. I haven't felt good for a couple weeks now. But lately, I've been miserable."

I think I'd finally convinced my friend. "Wow, what are you going to do?"

"I don't know," I said. "I've always thought any woman who had a pregnancy late in life, was just careless and stupid. Now I'm one of them."

My mind kept rejecting the information. Every time I tried to focus on the problem, I became overwhelmed. Ignoring it was getting me through the days. But I knew it was time to do something.

"I have an appointment with Dr. Curtis tomorrow. I'm going to wait and see what she says before I tell Hunter."

"Good idea," I heard Rose say. "I guess you will have. . .options?"

There was that sinking feeling again. My breathing became rapid and I felt like my heart was going to pound out of my chest. I couldn't face that question right now.

"I gotta go," I said, no doubt leaving my friend with more questions than answers. I dropped my phone into my purse and zipped it, as if I was burying the evidence. My hands were shaking and my last cup of coffee was in my throat. My third panic attack of the day was imminent.

I opened the back door and slipped out onto the porch. I gulped the air like it was sweet nectar. I folded my hands tightly and prayed this nightmare would be over. What was I going to do? My wonderful life, as of late, was falling apart. I never felt well anymore. I lived with a dull, continuous pain permeating my body. My thoughts were foggy and my memory was worthless. How could I have let this happen? Shouldn't I have known I could still get pregnant? Why didn't someone tell me? Why isn't it posted somewhere in life that you can still get pregnant at 51? I thought about crying but I'd done that already today. Being angry seemed the more responsible approach—but at whom? My husband? Myself? God? I shut my eyes and willed this whole mess away, knowing that wasn't possible. I had to deal with it—but not now. Now, everyone was hungry. I needed to focus on my duties as the mom and wife of a busy household. Letting them in on my little secret definitely wasn't going to happen today.

I took one more minute to give myself a private pep talk, then I went back to the kitchen and turned my thoughts to dinner. Although I hated to cook, and my stomach wasn't up for it, it was definitely more appealing than contemplating pregnancy woes. I opened up the freezer and waited for something to jump out at me. Nothing looked appetizing or easy-to-make. I toyed with the idea of just calling out for pizza, but that was my go-to on a busy school night. Instead, I picked up a bag of tater tots and a box of chicken. This would have to do.

I popped the frozen items in the oven and sat down at the kitchen table. My head hurt, my hands were trembling and I felt like I could throw up. I swallowed the bile in the back of my throat and allowed those pangs of worry to hit me again. I just couldn't turn off my thoughts. I tried to reassure myself that things would be fine. But, how would anything ever be 'fine' again? I already had 3 children—three *older* children! I counted out the months in my head of when this baby would arrive. January? February? The exact date didn't matter. It was the fact that there would be 15 years difference between it and my youngest child! My gosh! I was planning to retire in 6 years! I was old! I was tired! I couldn't physically handle a baby right now!

And Hunter. . .he would never be able to accept this news! He acted traumatized at the news of being pregnant with number 3! To tell him now, at his age of 55, and after all these years, I was expecting again? I don't think our marriage could survive it! I was so stupid! I stopped using birth control after my periods stopped. Obviously, I was still fertile! I gave myself another mental tongue lashing and felt the tears begin. My perfect life, my perfect life. . .what was I going to do?

I heard Callie, my youngest, close the garage door behind her. I quickly dried my eyes and prayed she wouldn't notice what a wreck I was. . .

Too late! I couldn't mask the embarrassment and concern on my face.

"What's wrong?" she asked the moment she saw me.

My thoughts jumbled in my mind. I didn't know what to say.

"Mom, what's wrong?" she asked again. "You look like you've been crying."

"Oh, no, I'm fine," I lied, still racking my brain for the reason. "I. . .I just pinched my finger in the drawer." The silly lie was the best I could do.

"Ooooh, let me see," my daughter said, being her usual considerate self.

"There's really nothing to see," I said, rubbing my finger. "There's no mark. It just hurts." I hoped my acting job was enough. I wasn't capable of coming up with anything better.

"Did you run it under cold water?" she asked. "That's always what you tell us to do."

"No, I'll give that a try," I said, thankful for the reason to turn my back toward her. I ran the perfectly fine finger under the water then quickly turned the attention to her.

"So, what's up with you?" I asked, pulling myself together mentally, as best I could.

"I'm going over to Connie's if that's okay. Her mom tried this new recipe and she invited me over for dinner. She knows I'll eat anything, and that I'll say I love it no matter what it tastes like."

I laughed at her reasoning. "You've had lot of practice with my dinners, right?"

"Awe, you're not as bad a cook as we always like to pretend. We just like to tease you, Mom."

"Thanks for the compliment. . .I think," I said, happy to have my mind on something else. Maybe that would be my saving grace tonight—staying so busy I wouldn't dwell on my problem. There would be plenty of time for that after my appointment tomorrow.

"You go right ahead and go," I said with a genuine smile. I'll think of you as we're enjoying our delicious meal of tater tots and chicken fingers."

"Oh, I picked a great night to miss!" Callie laughed. "I'll talk to you later. Leaving for Connie's!"

"I watched my daughter put on her light jacket and head out the door. Her best friend lived in our development. The girls grew up doing everything together. I'm glad they had each other.

I couldn't stop the next thought from entering my mind. I wondered who would be my new daughter or son's best friend? I started to mentally go through the houses down each street in our development, trying to remember if any of them had little kids. I never imagined I would be looking for new friends with small children at the age of 51.

I somehow managed to get my quick-fix meal on the table without another tear. I'd forgotten how easy it was to cry when you were pregnant. But, never fear, my hormones were ready to alert me to any tendencies I might choose to forget. It seemed like, with each passing moment, I recalled some distant memory from years ago, or felt a feeling reminiscent of those early days of pregnancy.

"This chicken isn't bad," Brint said, reaching for his fourth piece. I looked down at my plate. Mine was still untouched. I played with my tater tots, hoping no one would notice I hadn't taken a bite of anything.

"Eat up!" I chirped. My plate in my hand, I made my move to the sink. My stomach was dancing the rumba. Just smelling the chicken still on the stove made me queasy.

"Aren't you hungry, Mom?" Ann's question sent my brain on another search for words.

"Oh, I was grazing on snacks all day." My twenty-one-year-old looked at me, satisfied with my answer. She handed me her plate on the way to her room. She was doing her student teaching this semester, her last major hurdle before she became a teacher herself. It seemed like her every minute was devoted to lesson plans and preparing for upcoming classes. I was so proud of her. I knew she would make an excellent teacher.

"I'll clean up," my hubby announced. "I'll knock these dishes out, then I've got to head back outside." He'd starting cleaning up the yard after the harsh winter we'd had. There was plenty that needed done.

"Thanks," I answered. "I have some school work to do. I'll be out in a little while to see if you need help."

"I'm good," he replied. "You go get your school stuff done."

I was happy for the get-away opportunity. I left the room and made a bee-line upstairs. I always had something from school to do. I loved my life as a teacher, but with it came an endless scroll of must-do's and a never-ending stack of papers, just waiting to be corrected. Yes, there was plenty to do, and I would eventually get done. But right now, all I wanted was my pillow and some alone time. I needed to get my head back on straight and prepare myself mentally for tomorrow's appointment with Dr. Curtis. The school work would have to wait.

I shut my eyes and allowed those feelings of apprehension to return. I spent my time calculating due-date possibilities and wondering when and if I'd ever be able to retire. I closed my eyes, praying everything would be better after a nap.

My plan was to take a fifteen-minute break, then languish in a hot shower. After that, I would tackle the three piles of social studies tests I'd brought home to check, then get to bed at a reasonable time. My mind would be too busy to stress over tomorrow's worries.

I should have known better. There was no nap. Instead, I fell asleep—soundly. I awoke a little after 11 pm, just as my husband was ready to crawl into bed. After my few hours of rest, I was wide awake and wishing it was time for school. I took my shower as everyone else climbed in bed.

My mind was racing. For the first time in weeks, I felt energized. Even my spirits seemed to be lifted. The tears were gone, replaced by positive thoughts for the future.

So you're going to have a baby, I chided myself. What's the big deal? You've had three before. And it's not like you're eighty! You're only 51! Plenty of older women are having babies these days! And Hunter? He would just have to get used to the idea. After all, I didn't get pregnant on purpose. He would know that this was a total fluke! Maybe even a gift from God! Maybe this little boy or girl would grow up to cure cancer or become the president! Where was my faith? God had a plan for me! I would accept the challenge he gave me and be the best mom possible!

My little pep talk worked. I fell asleep with excitement in my soul—going over baby names and the joys that came with a new little one. I hadn't slept so well in years.

My good mood lasted into the next day. Despite the fact that I threw up whenever I smelled the cafeteria's lunch, the day with my students was enjoyable. I looked at each one of them in a new light. I was going to be a mom to a little one again! Instead of dreading telling Hunter my news, I made a list of silly, little ways to tell him. Baby clothes in the laundry? Coupons for diapers left on the counter? A bottle of mint ginger ale in the refrigerator, the only thing that settled my stomach when I was pregnant with our son? By the time my appointment came along, I was optimistic and ready to follow the regimen an 'older mom' would need to take on.

"So, this is a surprise!"

I took the doctor's words as a scolding.

"Yeah, a little," I lied.

"Well, babies aren't always planned," Dr. Curtis said. "It will take a little while for this to sink in, I'm sure." She paused. I nodded.

"Let's get the obvious questions answered first," she said, knowing I had to have dozens of things to ask her. "When is the first day of your last period? We'll get the due date and move on from there."

"Well," I said thinking back to that time in my life, "I am pretty sure it was February of 2009."

The doctor stopped typing notes and looked at me.

"You haven't had a period in over 3 years?"

I shook my head.

She flipped back through the folder she had in front of her. The quizzical look on her face made me a little nervous.

"Lisa, my records indicate you started through menopause around that time."

"I know," I answered quickly. "This is crazy. I never would have dreamed you could get pregnant after all that time. I thought I was done with menopause. I should have known better. There was no way I was lucky enough to get over this dreaded time so quickly. And now look where I'm at."

The look on my doctor's face was penetrating my entire being. Reality was kicking in. This pregnancy wasn't 'a fluke'. It was a little boy or girl forming inside of me. I had allowed myself to feel excitement and hope. Instead, I could be pregnant with a little one who would suffer with birth defects because of my ignorance and stupidity. This child may suffer its entire life due to me. I could feel a tear trickle down my left cheek. I was torn between crying and, dare-I-say, laughing, at the absurdity of it all.

"Dr. Curtis, this has really caught me off guard. My husband is gonna freak out," I said, leaning more on the side of crying now. "My older children might resent me. This whole thing has me. . .has me. . ."

My brief encounter with excitement had ended. The tears flowed freely now. My life was falling apart.

"I mean, am I too old to be a mom again? Is the baby going to be okay? I'm 51 years old! I know the chances of Down's Syndrome are higher, and there are other risks I'll have to be concerned about. And I know you are going to hit me up with the suggestion of aborting. I don't even want to talk about that right now." Another round of tears took over.

"I'm rambling. I'm sorry," I said, reaching out for the tissue Dr.Curtis was offering. "I'm sure you should be the one doing the talking. You are the one with all the answers. I'm just going to be quiet and let you talk." I put my hand to my mouth, covering it like a little girl would when she wanted to silence herself.

"The doctor gave me a comforting smile.

"Lisa," she said, it's going to be okay. I've dealt with many women in your situation. They've all survived." It was meant to make me feel better. I tried. I tried very hard.

"When did you take your pregnancy test?"

Not this again!

"I haven't taken one," I said. "I know what it's like to be pregnant."

The look on Dr. Curtis's face was blank. She stood up and turned to the cupboard above the sink. She took a box from the stack in front of her and handed it to me.

"We'll talk when you're done."

I watched the woman walk out of the room. I wanted to be mad at her condescending actions. Instead, I read the directions on the box and followed through with the test. When the doctor next came in, I was sitting on the stool crying. The negative stick was on the counter.

"What's wrong with me?" I asked between sobs. "I should be thrilled I'm not pregnant. And here I sit, crying!"

Dr. Curtis gave me a professional's hug and sat down on the chair in the room. I dried my eyes and waited for her to speak. I felt like an idiot.

"Well, we've ruled out pregnancy. That's the good news. I think you're having some mixed emotions over this, and that's perfectly normal. You've been trying to convince yourself for days that a new baby would be a good thing. Now you're trying to change your feelings in an instant. You've got to give yourself a little time."

I nodded my head. She knew exactly where my thoughts were.

"I knew you being pregnant was a highly unlikely possibility. But stranger things have happened."

I let her words sink in. "I guess it was pretty silly of me to think I could be. But my hormones are so out of whack. And I do definitely feel the same way I did fourteen years ago when I had my last baby."

"There are all sorts of reasons for your hormones being out of whack. We'll do some blood work and find out your levels. Then we'll know where to start. In the meantime, get yourself calmed down, and, Lisa, enjoy life at 51."

I smiled. I took a deep breath and allowed myself to feel a little happiness at the news I'd received. Life was going to get back to normal. I could live with hot flashes and moodiness. I had blown this whole thing out of proportion. Pregnant at 51? Seriously? What was I thinking? I usually wasn't one to jump to conclusions! But that's exactly what I had done. I had acted stupidly through all this. Maybe my hormones were clouding my judgement. Maybe I just wasn't thinking very clearly. Either way, I needed to put this embarrassing scenario out of my mind and move on.

I walked out of the doctor's office with a positive mindset. I just needed to relax and get my head on straight. I had a lot on my plate. I was busy! I was middle-aged! I would have aches and pains and strange things going on with my body. I would have stress with three children and a full-time job. I just couldn't panic when weird little things came up.

Fortunately, my busy lifestyle and demanding work schedule didn't allow me to dwell on this pregnancy scare for long. It was March—a busy time for a teacher of 4th graders. Spring break was coming and I had plenty to keep my thoughts occupied. I needed to finish my unit on the early settlers and get the students prepared for the test. It was also getting nice out. Spring had arrived early. Evenings would be spent outside, cleaning up winter's harsh mess, and preparing for the flowers and gardening sure to come. Along with those busy measures, my own kids were involved in all kinds of activities. And my husband had just committed to turning our basement into the family room he'd always promised me. Yes, my life should have been getting back to normal. Every day I expected the anxiety to fade. I anticipated life with my stamina back, ready to take on the world. I longed for my sharp memory to return. I was torn between worrying myself sick over my symptoms, and trying to forget about them. Nothing seemed comfortable anymore.

There was one thing I was adamant about, though. I could not let my family or friends know about my health concerns. I hated when people went on and on about their insignificant problems, seeking sympathy for little ailments. I wasn't a complainer, by nature. I planned to keep it that way. Deep down I felt there was something wrong, but I wasn't willing to give into it either.

I did learn that planning out my days and staying on a schedule helped me cope, at least with my fatigue. Occasionally, though, I had to cheat and let the day take me where it may. Today was one of those days.

"Chocolate—small please." Callie's request was no surprise to me. My youngest daughter always got chocolate ice cream when we came to The

Milky Way. "Oh, I see the flavor for the week is teaberry," my mom said, hiding her smile. "I'll have a small cone of that."

"I never would have guessed," I laughed. My mom loved teaberry ice cream. In fact, that was the main reason we were here. A Sunday afternoon in the springtime—you couldn't get much better than this roadside shop. It was our destination of choice. A nice visit to Mom's wrapped up by a trip to an ice cream stand that I loved clear back in my childhood. This was exactly what I needed. The rough week was over, and it was time to get back to life as I knew it. I still had some nausea, and I was brutally tired, but I had to chock these symptoms up to hormone changes and my body starting to slow down after years of mothering and teaching. I was fine, I just needed to push any doubts to the back of my mind and motor on.

"And I'll have a medium vanilla." I could feel my daughter's eyes on me.

"A *medium*?" she asked. "What happened to your diet?"

I laughed off her comment and paid the girl at the window. We went to the nearest open picnic table in the shade and settled in to eat our treats. Ice cream was my weakness. I had worked here summers in high school. I could still remember how I congratulated myself each day I made it through without a cone. But my daughter was right. A small cone today would have been sufficient. Actually, I should have skipped the delightful treat altogether. My weight was up—not just by a pound or two, but by a good ten pounds. My usual lean self was having trouble squeezing into my loosest jeans. And shorts? I didn't even want to think about shorts. For some strange reason, I was continually ravenous. I never felt full anymore, and my guilt wasn't enough to stop me. Had I been pregnant, this scenario would have been expected. Instead, I was giving in to cravings for no reason. My willpower seemed to be gone.

We downed our ice creams quickly. This 80 degree spring day was a little unusual in Pennsylvania, but welcomed by most after a cold and particularly nasty winter. Ice cream wasn't going to last long in this weather!

We talked to several people we knew while we sat enjoying the day. As a teacher, I was always off weekends. But usually I was too busy with my own kids and errands to spend an entire day doing nothing. I decided this was going to be one of those days.

I watched as my mother, newly retired from 43 years as a nurse, talked softly to one of her neighbors. She was no doubt giving her friend some advice. That was my mom's specialty. She always had an open ear for anyone, and she always gave the best suggestions for any problem that would come up. She was such a strong woman! My dad died of a stroke when I was only nine. My mom was left with 5 children under the age of eleven to raise on her own. She was so dependent on my dad that she didn't even know how to drive when he passed away! She called the driver's ed. teacher at the high school to give her lessons! Thank goodness she had her nursing degree and got hired right away at a nearby hospital. I can't imagine how awful that would have been for her. But somehow, Mom did it. We were lacking in money, but never in love. We were a close-knit family, struggling through some really tough times. But it's funny how they don't stand out in my mind now. All I can remember are the happy ones.

I hoped that I would always be the mom to my kids that she was to us. I had three wonderful children, and a husband around all the time. My times weren't rough at all in comparison to hers. So when I did have a stressful day along the way, I would remember my mom and her strength. A phone call to her usually got me right back on track.

And I was every bit as pleased with my own kids as she was of hers. I attributed it to my husband and I being actively involved in our children's lives. Well, that, along with a little luck. Yes, you had to deal with what you were dealt in life. I grew up learning that. But being there for your kids was a gift no one else could give. As a teacher, I'd worked with children from all kinds of families. Some of the happiest kids I'd ever met were from the poorest of homes. Their pride in family kept them going. Their riches were in warmth and love.

We sat so long at the picnic table just talking to friends and some of my former students, that I was ready to order another cone. Instead, I convinced my mom it was time to leave. I ignored the little voice in my head reminding me I was growing tired. Instead, I took my mom back to her house and dropped her off. She laughed as she got out and told me she had enjoyed herself so much at the Milky Way, she was going inside to get her car keys, then drive right back. I was happy for her. My energy level paled to hers.

"You go, girl!" Callie teased as she waved goodbye to Grammy. I tooted the horn and we started the half-hour journey home.

Callie and I talked about the day and both agreed it had been a relaxing afternoon. My daughter then busied herself on her phone, leaving me to my think about dinner. I called my husband, hoping he would find the idea of eating take-out a good option.

"Too late for that!" he said cheerfully. "I already have burgers on the grill, a salad made, and a pan of brownies in the oven. We'll eat when you get here."

I smiled. *That* was why I loved this man! He was considerate and always thinking of ways to make life easier for me and the kids. The thought of hamburgers on the patio put my mind in a happy place. I secretly hoped he put two burgers on for me.

I let my mind drift to tomorrow. It would be the start of another busy week. I didn't mind, though. In fact, I preferred it. I wanted to be productive and inspirational to the students I taught. The need to teach was inborn in me, as much as my blue eyes and blonde hair. I taught for 8 years before Hunter and I started a family. I considered every one of those little ones in my class each year my own. I missed them in the evenings, and worried about them over the weekends. I tried to be their daytime 'mom away from home.' That's how I wanted my own children to be treated in their schools—to feel safe, happy and loved.

And now, after working more than 30 years, I still had the same zest for teaching I had when I started. Of course, I didn't have the same energy as I did at 22, but who does? Everyone slows down as they age. It was my passion for the job that kept me going. Teaching for me was like breathing, eating, or sleeping. It gave me the fuel I needed to change lives and make a difference. I just needed to take care of myself and my love for the job would do the rest.

The remainder of the day progressed as it had started. I was content. I had convinced myself that any little thing that bothered me, was due to fluctuating hormones. My bloodwork result would show that. Everything was going to be fine. I would start feeling better soon. I just knew it.

And an uneventful weekend had been just what I needed. With three kids, that didn't often happen. Someone always had to be somewhere, or my days off were filled with laundry and cooking and catching up on schoolwork I didn't have time for through the week. This little break was needed!

When I finally crawled into bed that night, I mentally checked-off each child in my mind. Callie was already asleep. She had spent her evening studying for an algebra test she has been dreading for days. I made note of that fact and wanted to remember to wish her good luck in the morning. Brint, was still out. He was watching a baseball game with a buddy and didn't have a class until 10 tomorrow. I was glad he was having a good evening, but I knew I wouldn't soundly sleep until I heard him pull in the driveway. Please don't go into extra innings, I jested to myself. And then there was Ann. She was still awake in her room, cutting out paper squares and reviewing essays from Friday. But I could hear her softly singing along to her music. Yes, she was in a happy place too. My children were all noted and accounted for.

My husband had gone to bed a half hour before me and was sleeping soundly. These few minutes, as infrequently as they came, were always blissful to me. I knew where everyone was and I had no one to worry about. I could let my mind roam without interruptions. Tonight, I thought about my mom and my family and how I was living the life I'd always imagined—even better! Not only was I a teacher with a wonderful family, I had achieved a goal I'd dreamed about since I was six years old. I was a writer—an actual author with books published! My first was a parenting guide for parents of preschool children. Being a teacher and a mom, this book of advice and activities came naturally to me. My second book was an adult fiction whodunnit. From there I went on to write several children's books. Of course, I wasn't famous, nor was I making enough money to quit my day job. But the feeling of putting down words that someone else would actually want to read was thrilling. Granted, I was teaching full-time and raising my kids in the midst of it, but I tried to find time every day to work on my 'projects'. My husband dubbed my minutes in front of the computer as my therapy time. He was right. Writing had always given me a rush that nothing else could, second only to teaching. Mixing my two loves together made for some wonderful stories. Earning a little extra on the side was just a bonus. Of course, I aspired to be on the Best Seller's List, but for now, this 'hobby' pleased a part of my soul with just the right warmth.

I spent my remaining minutes awake thinking about tomorrow's school day, my students, and the active week I had ahead. I fell asleep, content with my life the way it was.

The next morning, I woke with a splitting headache. My joints ached and I felt lousy all over. Hormones, I reminded myself. Hormones. I thought of calling in sick, but remembered, through the fog and pain in my head, it was the day my fourth graders were starting their history projects. That's not a job I would leave for any substitute to tackle. I dragged myself from the covers to the closet to the bathroom. My energy was beyond low. I even fell once! I sent up a silent prayer of thanks that I didn't get hurt. I lent an ear to the rest of the family, hoping they were all awake and moving about. As far as I could tell, it was just another normal morning for them. That's just the way I liked it—normal. I hoped that for myself today, right after I got rid of this headache.

My aches and pains did fade throughout the hours—probably because I had no time to acknowledge them. They melted into the back of my mind, overtaken by popsicle stick forts, essays on log cabin life, and every pioneer tool imaginable, from butter churns to anvils. I typically love these kinds of days as a teacher. I become one of the children—excited, inquisitive. My classroom becomes a museum of replicas and reports. All the students have something to offer.

But the throbbing in my head got my sole attention again by the end of the day.

"Mrs. Church, Jason is taking all the glue!"

"I am not! I only used a little bit!"

"Guys, we only have a little bit of time left. Please let's share and be kind to one another."

For the most part, the children listened to my advice. They were actually behaving pretty well for the lax classroom environment of the day. They helped me tidy up and put away as best as ten-year-olds could. I finished the rest on my own after the buses left. The chaos of the day had totally overwhelmed me. I was beat. I tried to think back to this day last year. Was I this tired after that work day too? By 5:30 I could do no more. I stacked the rest of the art supplies, took 2 more aspirin, and left for the day.

I walked in the door at home, hoping to whiff the hint of some meal being prepared. Instead, I was greeted by my husband, Brint, and Ann, all of whom had this look of anticipation.

"Where are the subs?" Brint blurted, with a mixture of horror and hunger in his eyes—a typical teen-age boy.

"Didn't you bring Callie home with you?" Hunter asked, confusing me even more.

Ann noticed my fumble and stepped in. "Mom, I just talked to Callie a bit ago. I think the sub fundraiser is wrapping up. I'll run over and pick her up and bring our subs home. I'll stop and get some chips and Pepsi too."

I let Ann's words try to penetrate the steel bands encompassing my head. Fundraiser? Callie? Oh, no! I was supposed to be there right after school to help! I was sure she'd be upset. I gave Ann a look of gratitude and let her slip past me out the door. I played my headache card and headed for my bedroom. I stumbled just as I reached the door.

"You okay?" Hunter asked, following me upstairs.

"Yes, I'm fine," I sighed, exasperated with myself. "I have one of those headaches where you can't think of anything else in the world—just how bad it hurts."

Hunter gave me the soft fuzzy blanket I kept on the chair in our bedroom. "Lie down for a bit," he said, sympathetically. "I'm sure you had a long day."

I smiled, my head making the decision for me that I wasn't going to talk. I eased myself onto the bed. My eyes closed as my head touched the pillow.

The next two hours of solitude fixed me up. My headache left me in a little bit of a haze, but the pain was dulled. I ate a sub with a generous portion of chips alongside it.

"I thought you were coming to help out?" I knew those words of Callie's were coming. I was prepared.

"I'm sorry, sweets," I said, feeling like I'd totally let her down. "I had such a busy day. I didn't think you'd mind if I skipped out on you this one time."

"No, that's fine," Callie answered, obviously not upset. "But you could have called to let me know. I would have gotten a ride home with one of the girls. I was waiting around a pretty long time."

"I'm sorry," I said, feeling that pang of pain only a parent feels when she's let her child down.

I allowed her to fill me in on her day and the little details of the sale I'd missed. I cut off another piece of a sub and poured myself some soda. I could feel the stress dissipating. Within fifteen minutes, I felt like my old self.

The next few weeks at school were busy ones.

"How many years till I can retire?" I joked with Hunter one evening as I was literally falling into bed. "The good news is, I *am* getting caught up at school."

"So soon?" he laughed.

"Well, let me see, I've graded all the projects. That is an accomplishment on its own. They are lining the halls, thanks to my aide, waiting for the parents to see them tomorrow afternoon. Thursday and Friday, I will have them work on their essays while I catch up any kids who didn't get done. Oh, there never seems to be enough time for this unit." My groan was more for me than for effect.

"And then?" Hunter asked. "Smooth sailing to the end of the year?"

I laughed. "I wish! The stacks of paperwork on my desk are practically piled to the ceiling. How I'm supposed to get through that and be ready for the end-of-the-year meetings is beyond me. The amount of social studies I have left to cover. . .it's turning my stomach just thinking about it."

Bravo! I had at least 'talked' like I was hanging in there. In reality, I was a mess. My headaches returned, day after day. My body ached like I had the flu. I was nauseous on and off, and my every step felt like a chore. My days were exhausting. I prayed every morning that I would just get the day off without a hitch.

Could it really be hormones making me feel like this? I scolded myself for doubting my diagnosis. But I couldn't imagine every woman felt this bad at menopause. If so, middle-aged women around the world would stage a major shutdown on life until they felt better. I just was being a baby about all this.

"Did you submit your grades?" a fellow teacher, whose name I couldn't remember at the moment, called out the friendly reminder as she passed my door the next afternoon.

I didn't answer.

Who was that? I'd worked with this woman for thirty years and I couldn't recall her name? What was wrong with me? Yeah, my brain felt foggier than usual today, but there was no excuse for not remembering a friend's name! The worst part though, was realizing I had NOT submitted my grades! The lurch in my stomach was like a punch once I'd realized my mistake. Of course, third marking-period grades were always due at this time. How can I have just forgotten about them?

I quickly turned to the grade book system we used on line, praying I would somehow find the grades all tallied and ready to go. Instead I found an incomplete spreadsheet. Random grades were missing, and of the ones there, the totals were way off. I had a number of students who were, according to my prior calculations, failing my class. I took a deep breath and planned my next action.

My phone call to the office was embarrassing.

"I'm having some computer problems," I said in my best lying voice. "What time do grades have to be in?"

"Four o'clock like always," the secretary said in, what I perceived a condescending tone.

"I'll do my best!" I whispered.

I glanced at my watch. I had twenty minutes to somehow fix this train wreck of a mess in front of me. I began filling in blank spaces, randomly at first, just giving the students the benefit of a doubt. But I quickly realized the disparity of it all. Just because I had no record of grades for certain students didn't mean I should empathize and give them A's. It wasn't fair to the others. I thought for just a moment.

"Screw it!" I said out loud, not caring if I was heard. "All of these kids are nice and most of them do exactly what they are supposed to do. I'm giving them all A's."

I went down through the document, filling in grades here, changing them there, until every one of my students had earned somewhere between 90–100%. I pushed 'submit', picked up my tote bag, and headed for the door.

I don't think the significance of what I did hit me till I got home. I HAD FORGOTTEN TO DO MY GRADES!! What was wrong with me? How could I have missed such a crucial step in the marking period? My stress level was at its highest today. My job was, once again, being extremely affected by my health. But why? The tiredness I felt in my bones was screaming the answer. Yes, my fatigue was really interfering in everything I did. I usually stayed after school for a little while each day the week before grades were due. But, in this case, I had been too tired to even think about staying any longer than I had to at work. I literally felt too exhausted at the end of the day to even contemplate another task.

It was imperative I figured out why I still wasn't feeling any better. It made sense with the pregnancy scare, and even with the idea of mixed-up hormone levels. But my bloodwork Dr. Curtis ordered came back normal. She just chocked everything up to overworking. I wasn't satisfied with that assumption. My fatigue wasn't "Boy, I'm tired. I had a long day." It was more like "Is it safe for me to drive a vehicle or make something on the stove with the way I'm feeling?" It was scaring me! No, terrifying me! I needed to know what was wrong!

The next morning on my way to work, I noticed the chiropractor in town had out a new sign. "Try body adjustments for chronic fatigue syndrome." I'd heard about that illness before, but never really investigated it. When I got to school, I googled the ailment. I read over the basics of it quickly. My heart fluttered as I read the list of symptoms—fatigue, sleep problems, headaches, anxiety, muscle pain. They might as well have had a picture of me standing there next to the list. It was me to a T! I made an appointment for that afternoon.

The more I read, the more elated I became! Chronic Fatigue Syndrome had to be what I had! Better yet, chiropractic adjustments would be a quick and easy fix! I breezed through the rest of the day, feeling comfort in what I had learned. I couldn't wait for my appointment. Things were actually going to get better!

The visit went well. Dr. Delamar had a wonderful bedside manner. He let me ramble on and on about my symptoms. And the adjustment he gave me actually made me feel better immediately. I had so much tension in my neck that he wondered how I was even doing my job! I walked away from the place with a better range of motion, a feeling of confidence, and an appointment card for next Thursday. I was the happiest I'd felt in weeks!

I welcomed the little break Easter brought us. A few extra days off school were exactly what I needed. I knew I would be able to relax and focus on family instead of history books and projects. And the chiropractor visits were working! I was actually feeling more relaxed and a little less tired.

I was ready for the holiday! My family always spent Easter Sunday at Mom's. By the time all five of us siblings got to her house with our kids and spouses, her home was packed.

Although my brothers and sisters all lived in the immediate area, I felt I never got to see them enough. Everyone was busy with their jobs and their own kids. Holidays became a time to reconnect and remind us of all we had to be thankful for.

My sisters, Glenda and Wanda, were both a few years younger than me. They were just a year apart. They were as close growing up as any sisters could be. Now they worked in the same doctor's office and lived only a few miles from one another. They each had two children. It was sometimes hard to remember which kids went with which mom. They were always together and seemed every bit as close as their mothers when they were young. I had to work at not being jealous of them. I lived 30 minutes from Wanda and 45 minutes from Glenda. I couldn't possibly hold a candle to what they had together.

Ty was my younger brother—we were just a year apart. In years past, he had become, the most sought-after bachelor in our area. But within the past few years, he had married a school teacher and became the dad of two children. His happiness was obvious any time you looked at him. He was an hour's drive from me, so I counted on holidays to catch up on his busy life.

John was the only one older than me. He was married to a reporter for the local news. He had a son in law in school and was busy as a state senator here in Pennsylvania. He lived twenty minutes from me, but being a politician, he was always in the news. It wasn't hard to keep track of him.

I looked around the table. Family, to me, was incredibly important. If it took holidays to bond us, that was okay. We made those days special and worked to keep in touch as much as possible in between. That had become more and more of a project for me lately—contemplating all of our favors. I even thought about writing some articles and possibly a book on the importance of family. It was weighing heavily on my mind for some reason. Perhaps it was the rebirth that spring offers, or maybe it was just seeing how quickly all the children in our families were growing. Whatever it was, I found myself dwelling on it more and more.

"Hey, remember the Easter egg hunts we used to have in the yard when we were kids?" The question from my sister, Glenda, sent my mind to wandering. Everyone else in the room laughed, recalling stories of finding the most or hiding them in the best places. It was a little disconcerting to me that I couldn't conjure up a single egg hunt. But I chocked it up to my new ailment, and pasted a smile on my face and laughed with the others. I'm overworked, I told myself. I have Chronic Fatigue Syndrome. It's not a big deal to forget some things from a long time ago. Don't worry about it. There was plenty else to talk about. Those thoughts got me through the rest of the day.

Life moved on. By mid-May, my thoughts of excitement for, and anticipation of, summer break were usually in full swing. But this year, things felt a little different. Despite the wonders the chiropractor was doing for my mood, my symptoms persisted—even increased. Evening naps were a must. My house and classroom had post-it notes with reminders everywhere. My aching joints made every job a major chore. Once again, it felt like every direction in my life was losing ground.

At work, the end-of-the-school-year fair was just a week away. I had been in charge of it since we started the event about ten years ago. I knew today it was high priority that I dig the banners out of the hall closet, and make an agenda for the games and activities. I couldn't put it off any longer. Usually, I had everything under control by this time.

I hustled to the hall closet after the students left the next day, getting there just in time to see a few other teachers walking away with the boxes of preparations for the fair.

"Hey!" I said, trying not to sound accusatory. "Where are you taking the supplies?"

The group looked at me and then at one another.

"You can join us," Mary said, struggling to balance the box she was carrying. "We have everything sitting out in the cafeteria. We're staying for a couple hours tonight to tie up loose ends."

"Well, that's always been my job," I said, more to myself than them.

"Mrs. Strong told us we were to take over this year. She said you were really busy these days."

"And we all thought it would be a good idea," Brittany said. "Remember what happened at conferences when we left you in charge."

The trio giggled. I was mortified. I had no idea of the things they were talking about. I only knew my principal and co-workers must be thinking I am incapable and perhaps even, incompetent. I'd never entertained such notions before. I didn't know how to react. I turned around to go back to my room before the tears began.

The wonders of the chiropractor visits became over-rated in my head. I did feel some better, but my overwhelming tiredness had returned. Perhaps it never really left. Maybe I wanted to feel better so badly that I willed my symptoms away for a while. It didn't matter. Whatever my problem was, it was back.

The next day, I cancelled my scheduled appointment with Dr. Delamar, and decided to use my time differently. I hoped for a good day. But my morning started out unusually rough. My drowsiness, on this particular morning, actually made it tough to endure the thirty-minute drive to work. Even with the window open, my eyes were heavy. I fought with myself to stay awake. Little sleep through the night contributed to my usual tired self.

Shortly after arriving at work, my head started to pound. I had too much to do at this point in the year to let things go. I had to muddle through. Although I'd realized my co-workers could successfully take over any situation I found difficult, I still hated the fact they felt the need to do it. In actuality, they had been doing it all year. I just hadn't noticed.

By the time the students boarded the buses that day, I was spent. I couldn't even imagine driving home. Maybe a candy bar would give me some energy. I forced myself to the faculty room and to the vending machine. I was trying to decide between a Snickers and Hershey bar when I heard my name over the loud speaker.

Instantly, my heart began to race. I could tell by the tone of the principal's voice on the intercom she was provoked. What did I do? Better yet, what didn't I do? She never seemed pleased with me lately.

I hastened my pace to the office. My breathing was growing shallow. I was in no mood for a fight. I'd made it through the school day. I just wanted to pack up my things and head for the door. I took a deep breath, promising myself I would not be argumentative.

"Please sit!" The command put me even more ill at ease. I moved to the padded chair across the desk from the woman.

"I've had a parent complaint about you, Lisa."

I let out a nervous laugh.

"About what?"

"It seems you have been writing remarks on students' test papers. There is at least one parent who has taken offense to this." She gave me her "explain now" look.

I had been a teacher for more than 30 years. I'd had my usual share of concerns with parents, but saying something offensive on a ten-year-old's test paper? No way.

"I don't know what you're talking about, Mrs. Strong. I do write annotations on their tests occasionally, but I can't imagine I wrote something insulting."

The older woman leaned forward in her chair and handed me a student's paper. "Fuck you! You're Lazy" was scrawled across the top in red ink. I nearly fainted.

"Is this your handwriting, Lisa?"

I stared at the words. It didn't look like my handwriting, but then my writing had been changing over the past few months. I attributed my sloppiness lately to the inconsistent quivering in my hands from being so tired. But still, to make a comment like this one—I couldn't own that.

"Mrs. Strong, I don't swear. I don't tell students they are lazy. And I certainly wouldn't lie to you about it. I did not write this. It has to be a student clowning around." I prayed my words would convince her.

"I believe you, Lisa. Still, I would appreciate if you call the parent when we're done here and tell her we've met about the issue. We will do everything we can to find this prankster."

I nodded. I picked up the test and left her office. Unbelievable! A parent actually alleged I would do such a thing?

Back at my classroom, I sat at my desk and positioned the test in front of me. I stared at it. I closed my eyes and wrote the same message at the bottom of the test. They matched. I was instantly sick. I could feel the blood rushing from my head, and the hard pit form in my stomach. I grabbed the trash can by my desk and threw up.

My mind racing, I concentrated hard, hoping to focus on the details surrounding this test. I vaguely remembered checking the papers on my bed as I watched the evening news. My head hurt and I was sleepy. Could I have heard something on TV and subconsciously written it down?

I put my head in my hands and let more tears flow.

Something was wrong.

Up until now, I had covered up my shortcomings fairly well, or at least I thought so. But it was getting harder. My mind playing tricks on me was another thing. I was starting to get scared.

"Lisa, are you okay?"

It was Marcy, the fourth grade teacher in the next classroom. She must have heard me crying.

"Lisa?" she said again. "What's wrong?"

I didn't know what to say. It was like I couldn't think fast enough. Should I lie to her, tell her everything was hunky-dory? Or should I confide in her about writing on a student's test? Thoughts crowded my mind. Would she tell others about me? Would she accuse me of being unfit? Would she laugh at me? Would she think I was neurotic?

It startled me when Marcy started walking toward me. I couldn't deal with this now. I hadn't the energy or the clarity to hash things out.

"Oh, I'm fine, I'm fine!" I lied in my most convincing voice. I stood up, hoping she would stop where she was and turn around. "I have a really bad headache and I just remembered I have a meeting tonight and Callie has to be somewhere and—you know how things get. Today, it's just all getting to me."

Marcy stopped half way in. I picked up a pile of papers and pretended to be busy packing my tote.

"Oh, I'm sorry. Is there anything I can do. . .?"

Her words were cut off by the buzz of my phone. I dug for it in my purse as I continued to convince my co-worker I was fine.

"Oh, it's the kids," I said, glancing at the phone. "I have to take this. Thanks for checking on me though. I'll be fine."

"Sometimes a good cry is all it takes," Marcy said. I put my phone to my ear and waited for her to leave the room. I answered the phone with a terse 'hello.' I didn't recognize the number of the caller. I prayed it was just some car salesman wanting to sell me a car. It wasn't.

"Hi Lisa," the voice responded. I knew I had heard it before but I couldn't have told you who it was for love nor money.

"Uh, hi, can I help you?" I stammered, starting to unpack my tote of the same erratic items I had nervously filled it with a minute ago.

"Yes, this is Dr. Fall's office." My mind raced. Dr. Falls?

"Are you coming to your dental appointment today?"

"Today?" I said, trying to sound busy. "I'm sorry, I didn't realize it was today. Can I reschedule?"

"Lisa, you've missed your last three appointments. We worked you in special today at your request. Is there a problem we don't know about? Are you avoiding coming here? It's just for a routine cleaning."

My heart sank. I could vaguely remember having this discussion before.

"Oh, I'm sorry," I said, "I really can't make it today. I'm. . . I'm not feeling well." It was the truth. I was in no mood to go to the dentist and chit chat about everyday things while somebody cleaned my teeth. I had bigger problems going on.

"Please tell Dr. Falls I am so sorry to keep missing my appointments. I'll call back and reschedule for a day I'm sure I can come."

The woman hung up. I didn't know if I had convinced her or not. It didn't matter. I did miss the appointments! I did write on that test! I did sit and bawl like a baby after trying to convince my principal I wasn't a bad person! There is something terribly wrong!

I'd been denying my onslaught of memory issues. If I had been a lawyer or a doctor, covering up such memory problems wouldn't be possible.

I would have lost my job by now. The only thing keeping me sane was my passion for teaching, My actions and words were automatic. I didn't need to think about writing prescriptions or meeting with clients. My love for the students and my years of experience allowed me to keep going. It was second nature.

I sat back down at my desk and went over the last couple of weeks in my head. I'd been like a different person! Could I really be suffering from some serious medical condition? Maybe I never did have Chronic Fatigue Syndrome. Could I be schizophrenic or have a personality disorder? Hormones and stress couldn't be causing these drastic differences I was just now seeing. It was almost like there were two me's. The one 'me' works my tail off and acts like Supermom, and the other 'me', who I don't even recognize, writes nasty things on students' papers, ignores deadlines, and forgets about her own kids! Was I having a breakdown of some sort? Maybe I was going crazy! Unfortunately, I didn't have the time or the energy right now to evaluate. Researching symptoms or seeing a doctor weren't options with the schedule I had. I was too busy with my own kids and end-of-the-year school activities. I could barely stay awake through supper these days, let alone take on the task of diagnosing myself. Whatever was wrong with me was going to have to hide itself a while longer.

I packed up my bag, for real this time, and headed for my car, with the nagging feeling I was forgetting something. I left the test on my desk and the whole incident behind me. Little did I know what darkness lay ahead.

I walked through the small parking lot, searching for my car. The buzzing phone in the bottom of my purse vied for my attention once again.

"Hello?" I fumbled with the keys as I balanced the phone on my shoulder. It was Callie.

"Hey Mom, how was your day?" she chirped, calming my initial reaction that I'd forgotten her again.

"Oh, it was great!" I lied. "I'm leaving now," I said, throwing my school bag and a mound of unchecked tests into the passenger side.

Ok, I won't keep you. I just wanted to tell you I got an A on my test!"

"Terrific!" I said, not really remembering what test she was talking about. But I was pleased, nonetheless.

"I'll tell you about it later," she said. "Be careful driving!"

I smiled as I put the phone down. Callie was my little worrywart—she kept track of who was where and what was going on. She was a fireball, spunky and passionate about life. School and cheerleading consumed most of her days, but she loved both of them.

I pictured Callie in her uniform. Her looks matched her personality. Her muscular build from tumbling lessons and cheer practice made her weight-conscious. She dreamed of looking glamorous. And her hair! The poor girl worked every morning to get her wavy long hair to cooperate. It, like her, had a mind of its own. She would style, braid, pin up, and straighten, never quite achieving those perfect results. She was adventurous and loud and always made me smile. Talking to her always brightened my day. And right now, it made my head hurt a little less. In fact, I'd forgotten all about the panic attack I'd just had inside.

I started my Honda and looked at the gearshift. It appeared foreign to me, for some outlandish reason. I couldn't remember how to put my vehicle in reverse! I stared at the letters before me: PRNDLL. The only thought that came to mind was a memory from high school. My driver's education teacher, the same one who taught my mom to drive, had given us a little trick to remember the order of the gears. Pe-rin-dool. I could hear his voice so clearly that I looked around to see if he was nearby.

"Pap?" I called out, remembering the nickname all the kids gave him. "Pap?" I opened my door and called for him one more time. The fact that he had died 15 years ago never dawned on me, despite my attending the funeral with a small group of friends.

I closed my eyes. An image of the former teacher appeared in my head. As if in a trance, I focused my attention on him, I noticed he was slowly decomposing. His face was melting away. His blue eyes had turned red, and blood dripped down what was left of his cheeks. A terror grew inside me like I hadn't known since I was a child. The image was now almost unrecognizable.

"Go away! Go away!" I put my head on the steering wheel. The hot leather burned my forehead. Why wasn't this car moving? I needed to be somewhere! The sweat trickling down my face jarred me back to the present. I gasped, as if unable to get my breath. It was so hot...so hot! I fumbled with the window control and gulped in some air. Had I fallen asleep? I know there were more cars here before! My whole body was wet and clammy. My head, once again, throbbed, this time to the beat of the radio.

I fumbled with the air conditioner and, without having to think, put my car in reverse. It knew its way to the road.

By the time I got to the center of town, I had forgotten the matter had ever happened. The buzzing of my phone once again, brought me fully back to reality. My husband's voice shifted my thoughts to home.

"Hi," I answered. "What's up?" I sounded like I hadn't a worry in the world.

"Where are you?" he asked with concern in his tone. "I thought you'd be home by now."

"Sorry," I uttered, my mind racing for an excuse. "I was checking tests and I—"

His words cut me off.

"It's okay," he said. "The kids are just getting hungry for their pizza."

"I'm just pulling into Domino's," I lied. "Need anything else?"

"Just you," he said. I smiled as I put down my phone. Hunter was the best! He always knew just what to say to make me feel better. We had been married 32 years and I didn't regret a moment. Times weren't always rosy, but we got along wonderfully and truly loved one another, even after all these years.

The pep talk I gave myself was stirring. I reminded the inner-me, as I did every day, of all my splendid joys. I also vowed not to let today's issues get me down. Focus on your family, I kept telling myself. My thoughts shifted again, this time to pepperoni pizza and a cold drink. Everything was going to be okay. It was if I had flipped a switch, turning myself back into the old me.

Fragments of the day floated through my mind like a puzzle as I drove home. I took the exit home, trying to shrug the day off. When I got to the stop sign, it was the strangest thing. I didn't know which way to go. This is crazy, I thought to myself. How could I get lost on my way home? I'd driven this way for years! I made a right and followed the road to the red light. I should have gone left back there, I realized. This is ridiculous Lisa! Get your mind on what you're doing! I made a right back onto the highway, downplaying this strange incident in my mind. I drove about a half mile and saw my exit again. I took it, scolding myself for being so stupid. And yet, when I got to the stop sign, I again became confused and made a right turn. I was lost.

I pulled off to the side of the road and pulled out my phone. By this time, I was trembling and crying. I choked back sobs when Hunter answered my call.

"I don't know where I am!" I cried. "I was driving and I got lost and. . ."

Hunter's soft voice and words of understanding helped me calm down. I wasn't aware of the alarm I must be causing him.

I took a deep breath at his request, and described to him the places around me. Within minutes, I was back on track and just moments from home.

As I pulled into the driveway, I dismissed the horrendous situation I had just come from. It was gone from my brain. But I did have a nagging feeling something from work was bothering me. That damn history test! I caught myself swearing again. What was going on with me? When I got out of my vehicle, I knew my face matched the sick feeling I had in the pit of my stomach. I put on a smile and told myself again—focus on your family!

The pizza was hot. The salad was ready. The soda was cold. Hunter did a wonderful job of hiding the scare I'd put into him. For the next twenty minutes my family actually sat down and had a meal together. I was enjoying the stories and conversations until I had this overwhelming urge to lie down. I stood up, unsure if I could even make it without help to my bedroom.

"Are you okay, Mom?" Callie asked. I almost didn't hear her. Her voice sounded so far away.

"Just tired," I murmured. "I'm going to relax for a little bit then I'll be back down."

I couldn't tell if she bought my excuse or not. I made my way to my bedroom. I practically fell onto the bed. I was too tired to think, or, even to recognize, my family was downstairs discussing me. The clinking of dishes and silverware being washed lulled me to sleep.

"Something's up with Mom," Hunter said, in a calm, but worried tone.

His three children looked at him, not very surprised at his words.

"What do you mean?" Callie asked. She agreed with her dad's comment but wondered what he had noticed different.

"Well, I think she's having some memory troubles," Hunter answered. He let the words settle before he continued. "Have you kids noticed anything a little off about her?"

Ann was the first to respond. "I have," she said. "She definitely is forgetting things. I didn't make a big deal of it at first, but I've noticed this more and more."

"Yeah," Brint added. "She just doesn't seem like herself. She's kind of like a subdued version of herself."

Hunter nodded while choosing his next words carefully.

"She called me on her way home from work. She didn't know where she was."

Ann gasped. Callie got tears in her eyes.

"You mean like Alzheimer's?" Ann's words were tinged with shock.

"I don't really know," Hunter said. "Her memory has been off, but you know, she's been so tired lately. Maybe she's overly tired and it's affecting her thoughts."

"Maybe," Brint said. "I have noticed, too, that she seems to be having some trouble walking. She runs into stuff a lot."

Callie was almost shaking at the notion of all this news. She anxiously added what she'd noticed.

"I saw her fall the other day."

"Where?" Brint reacted quickly to these words.

"She was getting out of the car last week. I thought she must have just lost her balance, but maybe there's more to it than that."

"I agree," Ann said. "What do you think we should do?" Her gaze at her father was full of concern.

"Well, I think we each need to keep track of anything she does that is troubling," Hunter replied. "Her naps, her words, her actions. . .anything we notice that is out of the ordinary."

"Should we talk to her about it?" Callie questioned the group. "Can't we just ask her what is wrong?"

"I don't know if it's all that simple," Ann conveyed in a hushed tone. "She may not even realize something is up. Let's just keep it to ourselves for a while."

The group nodded their heads, almost as if they were taking a silent vow. The secret was out. The entire family knew of the symptoms I was experiencing. Only time would tell if I was going to improve.

They cleaned up the supper dishes quietly, each one reflecting on his or her own thoughts. They were glad I was upstairs sleeping. Inviting me to the family meeting would definitely have been a mistake.

About 9:00 p.m., I felt a nudge. My eyes darted frantically about the room. By the time I noticed Callie, I was trembling.

"Mom, it's me," she said softly. "You've been sleeping all evening. Do you need to get up for anything?"

I sat up in bed, quivering like a frightened child. It took a few more seconds before I finally realized it was my daughter beside me.

"Oh, Callie, I'm sorry," I said, feeling embarrassed. "I thought I would just lie down for ten minutes. I never expected to do this. I'm sorry!"

"I've been waiting to talk to you all night," she said. "I thought you'd never come out."

"You should have come in," I teasingly scolded. "You know you can talk to me any time."

"Dad told us to leave you alone," Callie mumbled. "He said you weren't feeling good. He said you got lost on your way home from work."

I had totally forgotten all about that incident. It was then that I could see the deep creases of worry in her face. She left the room. I followed her down the hall and into her bedroom.

Callie plopped down on her bed. I scrunched in beside her, making myself cozy on her plethora of pillows. It was crazy, but even with my concern for her, I had to make a conscious vow to stay awake while we sat there.

"Talk to me," I said, putting my arm around her. What would it be this time? Boys? Homework? It was as if she had never uttered the words about me being lost.

"You're acting funny."

I didn't pick up on her serious tone.

"What do you mean?" I asked, reminding myself already to stay awake.

"You aren't acting the way you usually do." She paused, as if she were deciding what to tell me next.

"Did you go to the Cheerleader's Booster Meeting before school this morning?"

My heart dropped.

"You're the secretary, Mom! You have to go! You said you would! I reminded you last night!"

Panic and embarrassment took over my being.

"Alyssa said they didn't have the board minutes to go over. And you were supposed to bring the uniform samples along to show everyone!"

I kind of remembered promising to stop in at the uniform shop a few weeks ago, but that had totally slipped my mind. And the meeting? I thought I put a reminder on my phone! Did I dismiss it like I had so many other things these days?

"Damn it!" The words were out of my mouth before I could stop them.

"Mom!" Callie cried. "You're swearing!"

My daughter had never heard words like this come out of my mouth. I was brought up in a family where we went to church every Sunday, had great faith in God, and didn't swear. This definitely wasn't like me.

"I'm so sorry," I said, reaching out to give my daughter a big hug. She retracted before I could touch her.

"Mom, you can't keep pretending! You got lost today just a few miles from here! You're not right!"

Her words were a hushed scream.

"You keep telling us the same stories over and over. You act like you're listening to us when we know you're not! You keep wearing the same clothes over and over. You need to listen to me!"

Tears began to stream down Callie's face. "Honey, come here," I said, pulling her close. It was strange, but her words didn't penetrate. I heard them but they didn't alarm me the way they should have.

"I know I've been acting pretty kooky lately." I needed an excuse! Words I didn't plan spewed from my mouth. "Work has just been so stressful, lately. As soon as school is out, things will be totally back to normal.

There's nothing for you to worry about. Just hang in there with me, okay? Your old mom here is fine."

Callie wiped away her tears and nodded. Her look and pleading words devastated me. What had she seen over these past months? Did she notice my hands trembled too much to put on earrings? Had she seen me fall in the yard this morning, or in the hall the other day, or the kitchen last week?

I gave Callie one more hug, promising all was well. "Now get back to your books," I said, giving her one more squeeze before I left. She gave me half a smile and a whisper of thanks. All I could manage for her was an empty promise.

The next day was horrendous! My wasted time checking papers late last night had cost me. It was nearly 4:00 am by the time I went to bed. When I did get up at 6:00 a.m., I was in a fog. The day was going by in slow motion. As hard as I tried, I couldn't focus on anything. I was fumbling over students' names who I'd taught for the last nine months. I forgot it was my turn for recess duty and I accidentally locked myself out of my classroom. I needed a break.

"Enough is enough, Lisa." Rose's words got my attention. We were meeting for coffee after school—a rare treat for both of us.

"You have too much on your plate," Rose continued. She had listened to the secrets I hadn't told anyone else.

"This is not like you. Falling asleep at your desk? Trouble remembering things? It sounds like there could be something more to this."

A dozen thoughts entered my mind. Rose was not telling me anything I didn't already know. I guess I was just looking to her for some consolation that I was just too busy. But I wasn't getting that.

"Maybe you need to talk to someone," my friend said hesitantly. "Maybe your anxiety and strange thoughts are things you just need to share with someone. I'm a good listener, but I'm not a therapist."

I tried not to take offense at her suggestion. I didn't need a therapist! And yet, when Rose wrote a number on a piece of paper and handed it to me, I tucked it in my purse. I'll call tomorrow, I thought.

I let a few days go by before I gave the therapist another thought—not because I was avoiding her. . .but because I had totally forgotten Rose and I had talked about her. Giving my life a concentrated effort, as I had decided before, wasn't going to be enough to get me through the next couple of weeks. It wasn't fair to my family or friends. I needed someone to tell me I was normal. I needed reassurance. Then, I would be okay.

I took the next day off work, lying to everyone that I was plagued with a horrendous headache. By the time I got to the woman's office, it was no longer an untruth.

"So tell me a little bit about yourself," the woman began, trying to put me at ease.

I succumbed to her intentions, filling her in on my wonderful family.

"I'm not really sure why I am here." My words stumbled out of my mouth. "I really do live a pretty charmed life," I took a breath. I can do this!

"My husband, Hunter, is great. He's a teacher as well. That makes it really nice for us in the summer and on holidays. We have three kids—two girls and a boy, making our family the perfect one I'd always dreamed of. We made it through the early years with the kids easily. But now that they are older—ages 14, 18, and 21, each day is a new adventure. Thank goodness they are all good kids!"

I paused, worried that I was rambling. The therapist still seemed interested.

"Hunter and I have always worked hard to instill good values and morals in them over the years. I'm especially happy with their spiritual lives. I made sure the kids and I attended church and that they became involved in church activities from the beginning. I'm proud I could follow through on it alone. Uh. . .it just wasn't Hunter's thing."

The therapist smiled and wrote something down. I felt the need to continue.

"Sounds like you have quite the family, Lisa."

I smiled in agreement back at the woman.

"Yes, one would think my life should be perfect. But I'm having some strange things going on lately."

The woman listened intently as I described strange dreams and grizzly thoughts.

"I can't really explain my ridiculous nightmares," I said to the woman. "They have no main theme or repetitive manner. Some are scary, like me being lost in the woods, and some are terrorizing, like the night I dreamed 2 rapists broke into our home and took my girls and I away in their car. I woke up that night in tears, screaming uncontrollably. Thank goodness the kids slept through it. Hunter somehow managed to get me calmed down without too much consoling.

I told her of recent panic attacks and my forgetfulness. They were really wreaking havoc on my family time and school life.

"Yesterday I couldn't remember how to turn our washing machine on," I began. I turned all the buttons and pushed everything that should be pushed. I couldn't get it to work. I was too embarrassed to ask Hunter or the kids how to work it." I paused for a few seconds.

"This isn't normal," I whispered, tears now streaming down my face. "How can a mom forget how to do the laundry?"

The woman looked at me sympathetically. She had to think I was crazy. But did it really matter what she thought. I skipped any more examples and moved on to other things.

"My over-all health hasn't been that great either," I confided." I've fallen several times at school and at home. I'm not usually a clumsy person."

The woman took some notes and nodded her head. I guessed she wanted me to continue.

"I've also had a large increase in the number of headaches I get. Some are migraines, some are tension headaches. My life is really stressful right now. Being a school teacher at the end of the year is awful and I have 3 kids and. . ." I was rambling. I couldn't even tell if the woman was listening any more.

"And I'm so tired. . .always tired. I just can't wait to go to bed each night and I hate getting up in the mornings. I never have enough energy. I'm afraid my husband and kids will get mad at me." That last thought was totally ridiculous. I couldn't imagine how it even came out of my mouth.

I felt stupid as I regurgitated my list of symptoms. After hearing them all, I truly believed the woman would declare me certifiably crazy on the spot. Instead, we talked about my everyday life.

"I think you do have a good bit of stress in your life right now, Lisa," the counselor said. We can focus on these things on our next visit. We can talk about making life easier."

I nodded, feeling relieved that she believed me, but inept for not knowing how to make my life easier on my own. This wasn't something I needed to sit and talk about with someone.

For now, I'm going to give you some relaxation techniques that will help get you through stressful times. But I do want you to get some medical help for your headaches. You mentioned a migraine specialist earlier. I think you ought to make an appointment to update him. We spent the last ten minutes of my designated hour on how to breathe from my diaphragm and to recognize a panic attack coming on.

I left, not feeling particularly hopeful. I thought my problems were far beyond learning how to relax. I took the handout she gave me out of courtesy. I told her I'd call for my next appointment. However, I did think talking to my doctor about my headaches was a good suggestion. I vowed to take care of that soon.

I kept the therapy visit a secret from my husband. It wasn't that I was embarrassed, I was just too physically tired to even talk about it that night. At 10:00 pm, I sunk inside my covers, allowing the cool blankets to swallow me. I didn't care about school, or my kids or my husband. I just wanted sleep.

Most nights I slept soundly, not moving until the early morning alarm. But tonight, I slept for only a few hours, then woke on my own. My sleep had been fitful and riddled with a series of ridiculous dreams. Thoughts of bugs, rat poison, and rotting food swirled in my head. I glanced at the clock. 2:52. Any other time I would welcome the few more hours to sleep. But tonight, I just wasn't finding peace. My stomach was doing a number on me as well. Perhaps a trip to the bathroom would solve everything.

My bedroom was dark, but I had this walk down in my sleep. After getting up with babies over the years, I could get anywhere in the house blindfolded. When I bumped into the corner of my dresser, I chalked it up to fatigue. But when I stumbled in the bathroom—that was a different story. I veered right, guiding myself smack into the side of the tub. I spiraled and fell forward in a heap, face down in the sea of white. My head came within inches of slamming into the faucet. Instead, I felt my cheek hit the tub hard, sending pain through my head.

I lay there, expecting everyone to come running. I heard no one. Had I really fallen? Maybe this was just a dream. Sometimes people didn't check on you in your dreams. Maybe I was still in my bed, having a nightmare that I fell in the tub! I put my hands on the bottom of the tub and pushed myself up. I got to my knees. I couldn't think of anything to say. "Ouch," I finally mouthed aloud, deciding this fall warranted some kind of verbal outburst. I mentally checked my bones for aches or pains. I seemed to be okay. I sat in the dry tub for another minute or so, still thinking my husband or one of the kids would surely come check on me. With this gang, I could be here for hours, I mused. "Get up and get back to bed!" I commanded myself.

It was harder to stand up than I expected. My arms and legs weren't cooperating. I kept falling forward every time I tried to get up. Finally, I pulled myself out of the tub, holding onto the sides like I was climbing a mountain and coming down the other side. I felt like I had mastered a great feat simply by getting free of the porcelain monster. I found myself on the floor, braced against the toilet like I needed it for balance. Had I been drinking, I wondered. I felt so unsteady I couldn't imagine any other explanation. I tried to recall the last several hours. My mind was in a fog. My memory wouldn't penetrate the haze. I didn't remember going to bed or anything else from the day before.

My eyes finally adjusted to the darkness. The light of the half-moon brightened the bathroom enough for me to get my bearings. I grabbed the windowsill, pulled myself up, and turned around. To hell with my stomach, I thought. I needed to find my bed.

I took a deep breath and let go. Turning toward my bedroom, I took a few baby steps. My knee hit the bedpost as I grasped at the air. Why was I walking sideways? I entertained the thought of waking my husband, but what would I tell him? "Honey, I just fell into the bathtub and I can't find my way back to my bed—but don't worry, I'm fine." It was frightening enough to *me*. I couldn't imagine how he would feel.

I held onto the bed like a blind woman, feeling my way back to my pillow. I eased myself down onto the bed, and curled up in a ball. Despite my anxiety over the situation, I fell asleep in seconds. I woke the next morning in the same position.

Had I been dreaming? Was the nightmare over? I honestly didn't know if my strange mishap occurred, or if it had been some sort of night terror. I sat up slowly. My body felt normal. My head was clear. I walked into the bathroom and looked for signs of my fall—a towel on the floor, or the shower curtain dangling. Nothing seemed amiss.

"It was a dream," I breathed out loud. "All a dream . . .." Relief filled my soul.

I brushed my teeth and swished around a capful of Scope. A look in the mirror was necessary. I almost didn't recognize the face staring back at me. I had dark circles under my eyes. My wrinkles were no longer laugh lines as I used to joke. They were pronounced, firm, and noticeable creases in my face. I looked 10 years older than I was. I appeared tired, like I hadn't slept in days. Is this always what I looked like? I couldn't remember.

I brushed on some mascara and smoothed on pink blush. I ran my fingers through my hair and smiled back at my reflection. This was how I was going to present myself today. I wasn't going to dwell on the negative aspects of the last couple of months. Everything could be easily explained. The falls were my own fault for not being more careful. My memory lapses were normal for someone going through menopause. That was why women dreaded this time in their lives. And the episode last night? It was all a terrible dream. There was no reason to worry about anything. I just needed to start acting my age and taking better care of myself. There. A simple solution.

Two days later, I got into Ann's car with a smile. My headache guru in Pittsburgh had a cancellation. I took the therapist's advice and counted on him for some insight into my problems. I reluctantly filled my daughter in on my influx of falls and the worrisome memory issues on the way. She pretended to act surprised, but I knew deep down she was well aware of my condition. When the doctor finally saw us, she spoke first.

"Something's wrong."

Despite the fact we had rehearsed, Ann's words still startled me. The physician's assistant was taking notes.

"What do you mean?" Dr. Kifer asked. My daughter looked to me to continue.

As if on cue, I gave the doctor the run-down on what had become my life. The symptoms I forgot, Ann filled in.

"I'm only 51, doctor," I said, trying to make him understand. I can't believe this is all due to menopause.

Dr. Kifer sighed and looked back through my chart. "Let's see," he said. "You started coming here in 2002. First it was for your migraines, but I see that you also had a seizure, what. . .about eight years ago?"

My mind instantly went back to that awful day. It was a Sunday morning. Hunter and I were enjoying a rare morning out with no kids in tow. We joked about finally having a little time to ourselves, only to spend it shopping at Lowe's Building Supply.

"I'll get in line," I remember saying, taking over the cart. "You make sure we have everything."

I no sooner had taken a step when a grand mal seizure engulfed my being. Thank God, Hunter was close by. He broke my fall to the ground by putting his arms around me. I writhed on the floor, releasing my bladder as I did so. Finally, I stopped shaking. My husband grabbed my hand and called my name. Nothing. "I can't find a pulse!" a concerned customer whispered. My husband dialed 911. Within minutes, the medics were there. I was transported to the local hospital.

Now, years later, I was in the neurologist's office in Pittsburgh, reliving that horrible day.

"You had said I was probably having a reaction to the high dose of Nortriptyline I was on for neck spasms. You cut my dose in half and put me on Topamax," I reminded him.

"Yes," the doctor responded. "Topamax can be used both as a migraine prevention drug and as an anti-seizure drug. You've been on it ever since then, with no more seizures, correct?"

I hoped he wasn't going for this being related to what I had now. I didn't want more seizures.

"Correct," I answered. "But, I looked up Topamax one day. Memory issues can be a side effect." I waited anxiously for Dr. Kifer's reply, hoping for another simple solution.

"Well, that's possible," the gentleman responded. "Let's see, you are on such a low dose of Topamax, I doubt it could even prevent seizures. I think we can take you off of it and see if your memory improves."

I looked to Ann. She had such a hopeful look on her face. A quick and easy answer was welcome news.

We left the hospital in Pittsburgh and chatted most of the way home. I felt rejuvenated—like I'd been given a second chance! Finally, I could talk about everyday life instead of my health. It was a glorious day. I felt like a weight had been knocked from my shoulders. I could get back to family life as normal. I smiled. Finally, I thought, this whole nightmare will be over!

"Can you get the hot dogs out of the oven?" I asked Ann at the start of another hectic evening.

My oldest daughter sauntered from the sink to the stove, a puzzled look printed on her face. She opened and shut the oven door.

"There's nothing in the oven," she said, turning around to question me.

"Oh," I said quickly, realizing my mistake. "I meant to say get the hot dogs out of the . . . the . . . ."

"Refrigerator?" She filled in the blank that I couldn't manage on my own.

I nodded. I had played this word retrieval game all day. I couldn't seem to say anything right.

"I don't know why I can't talk today," I apologized. "My kids at school kept correcting me, too."

"Some days are just like that," Ann answered. "I do that myself sometimes."

I appreciated the kind words. But what I was experiencing today was not normal. If I did it once, I did it 20 times. By the end of the day it was becoming a joke with my fourth graders. To some it was even annoying.

"Can you finish up here, Sweetie? I need a few minutes."

"Are you all right?" Ann asked. I recognized that same worried look from before.

"I'm fine," I answered.

I passed my husband in the hall. "Everything's about ready. I'll be down in a bit! Start without me," I quipped, touching his arm in reassurance. He smiled and kept moving. I was glad he didn't stop me. I didn't have the strength or the patience for a conversation.

My bed welcomed me like a long-lost friend. The top of the comforter was squishy and cool on my skin as I melted into the vastness. I promised myself, as usual, I would only lie down for 10 minutes, knowing full well, in my condition, I had no say in the matter. My body responded only to my exhaustion.

I awoke at 10:00 p.m. to the sounds of my husband in the shower. I sat up, bewildered and confused.

When he came out, I planned to ask him what he thought was going on with me. Instead, he came over and sat down beside me on the bed. He took me in his arms and just held me.

Finally, he spoke.

"Lisa, I'm sorry, but I have to ask. Are you taking some kind of diet drug or something that would make you act so . . . so detached from everything?"

"You think I'm on drugs?" I spewed out in an unexpected outburst unlike any I had ever displayed before in our marriage. "You actually think I am taking something to alter my behavior?" I couldn't believe what my husband was saying!

"No . . . no!" he protested. "Lisa, I'm just trying to figure out what's up with you." All of a sudden, I was furious.

"So, there's something wrong with me, huh?" I spit out my words. My normal voice tone was gone, replaced with a new one—peppered with resentment and hostility. "I can't believe I am sitting here letting you talk to me like this! How dare you think of me as insincere and, worse, a damaged product?" My eyes filled with tears. My heart was racing and my breathing was off again. Almost instantly my mindset changed. What was I doing? I never spoke to anyone like this before, let alone my husband!

"I'm so sorry," I cried in the same breath as my condemnation. "I don't know what I'm saying." I felt hot tears stinging my cheeks.

Hunter moved toward me and once again put his arms around my trembling body. "I'm the one who's sorry," he whispered. "I'm just worried about you."

"I know," I said. "This will go away. I promise I'll slow down and take better care of myself." I hoped my words convinced him better than they did me.

"Get yourself ready for bed," he said softly. "We saved you some leftovers in the fridge."

I took a deep breath and allowed him one more hug. I could feel myself calming down.

I smiled my thanks and got ready for a shower. Rather than dwelling on the conversation we just had, I thought about the food waiting for me downstairs. I was starving. It seemed like I always was now. I used to be able to go from morning to night with very little food. I was just too occupied with life to take the time out to eat. But within the last several weeks, I seemed to have a voracious appetite I couldn't satisfy. Despite my busy lifestyle, I'd added close to 15 pounds, now, within a few months. I slowly began replacing my petite wardrobe with one of dress sizes I hadn't seen since I was an overweight teenager. Even though I was dragging, I made my way down to the refrigerator and warmed my plate. My kids were scattered elsewhere throughout the house, so I found myself alone in the kitchen. I ate my leftovers, then blocked out the day with cookies and milk. I had done just enough to make myself tired again.

When Friday afternoon of the last full week of school arrived, my co-workers and I were scrambling for ideas to make a hot spring day meaningful, but pleasurable for the students.

"We could do some kind of art project together," Sharon said.

"That would be pretty hard to do out in that room," Carly said. "And I have my art supplies packed away."

"Me too!" Linda said.

"How about a spelling bee?" Michelle asked.

"Or this?" I said, taking the movie case out of my closet.

We all agreed this would be the perfect solution. We situated the four classrooms of students in the large group instruction room determined to make the most of any free time. If we each took shifts, we could reward ourselves with time to prep our rooms for summer and check student assessments.

I sent my class behind the others and plopped down on my desk chair. I felt a small sense of accomplishment that I had settled our afternoon dilemma. I hadn't been much use to my fourth-grade team as of late.

I looked about the room. It was a mess. By this time of year, I usually had all paper off the walls, the books collected, and my plants safely at home. None of that had happened. In fact, my back wall was still covered in the penguins my students had made in February. I tried to make a decision about where to start. Instead, I put my head down on my desk and fell asleep.

I woke up just minutes before my turn to oversee the students. My sleep had been productive. I was more alert than earlier. But I had used all the free time allotted me for working in my classroom. Maybe I could get a little bit done after school. At least I should be able to stay awake through the movie now. That gave me some consolation. That had weighed on me all morning. I grabbed a stack of papers, my red pen, and my laptop to record the grades. I took a deep breath and headed for the group instruction room. I was more than ready to take a seat in the air conditioned, quiet atmosphere.

The students were hushed and absorbed in the movie. I moved toward the empty seat reserved for the lucky teacher playing watchdog. Before I sat down, I surveyed the crowd, looking for those few talkative students who always made group activities a challenge. I spotted them, and made a mental note. Now all I had to do was tune out the blare of the movie and get a few papers checked.

I put my things down on the table and took a step back from the chair. Oh great, I thought, here comes a hot flash. I could feel the heat spreading through my body. I wished I had brought the bottle of water I had been sipping in my classroom. These ridiculous 'menopause moments', as I liked to call them, overtook me at the strangest times. I hoped the kids wouldn't notice my reddened face or the tiny drops of sweat above my brow.

The next thing I knew, I was waking up in an ambulance.

"What happened?" I asked the medic leaning over me.

"You had a seizure. We're taking you to the hospital to get checked out."

My mind tried to pick up what had happened over the last 30 minutes. Why couldn't I remember anything?

"Where was I?" My question was genuine.

"At the elementary school. I guess you work there?"

My eyes filled with tears. The students! They saw me! Dear God, please let this be a dream!

In a matter of minutes. I was chugged into the emergency room where I was transferred to a bed behind a drab green curtain. I shut my eyes tightly, willing this ghastly scenario away.

"Mrs. Church," I heard a male voice say as the curtain swung around to expose me. "How are you feeling?"

"I'm confused," I said, trying not to panic. "Is my husband here?"

"I believe they called him, yes," he said looking over the chart. "It appears you had a seizure." His eyes met mine, looking for confirmation.

"I guess so," I answered, still unable to remember the incident. "Exactly what happened?"

Before he could answer, my husband appeared from around the corner. He hustled toward me. I grabbed him for dear life.

"I had a seizure," I sobbed, letting all my anxieties crescendo at once. "I can't remember what happened."

"It's okay," he said calmly. "It's going to be fine." He rocked me back and forth for a moment, trying to comfort the crying mess I'd become.

"I need to get a little information here," the doctor interrupted politely.

Hunter filled him in on my medical history over the last 8 years. The doctor listened intently and made a decision.

"I will give this Dr. Kifer a call," the ER doctor offered. "He probably will want to put you on something else since you discontinued Topomax."

Hunter and I nodded our approval at his suggestion. The doctor gave me a once-over and checked my vitals again before he called. When he returned, he had some semblance of good news.

"It certainly appears as though you must have some seizure problem that necessitates staying on meds. Dr. Kifer told me to start you on a low dose of Depakote. The dose will be increased slowly for a few weeks until your body gets used to it. He'll phone-in the prescription."

As much as it hurt to hear I had a seizure disorder, strangely, it was a relief to know. Perhaps it was as simple as starting a new pill. The medicine would keep me safe from having one again. We left the hospital optimistically.

It wasn't until we were almost home that I summoned up the non-medical consequences of having a seizure. I realized I wouldn't be able to drive for six months—Pennsylvania state law.

"Everything is going to be fine," Hunter said in his most consoling tone. "Consider how well things worked out last time."

I dredged up that incident of so many years ago. I had my license revoked for only a few months because I got my neurologist to petition it back from the state. My seizure, at that time, was thought to be caused by a high dose of medicine, and the state returned my license. But now. . .I knew I could never be so lucky this time. My seizures were now some kind of condition. No doctor would acquiesce on this one.

Images of my students flickered in my mind. I just wanted this day to be over.

When we finally arrived home, Brint was the only one there. I cringed at the thought of telling him.

"What's wrong, Mom?" he asked as soon as he saw my face.

"Your mom had a seizure today at school. She's okay," Hunter said quickly, trying to alleviate that strain of panic Brint already had on his face. "We just got back from the hospital."

The look my son gave me was a blend of disbelief and fear. He may have been 18, but he still felt the pain of a kid needing his mom. He put his head down.

"She's going to be fine," Hunter said for the umpteenth time.

I got up from the table and went to the bathroom. I could hear them talking from there.

"Fine? What the heck does that mean?" I heard Brint ask. "Back to her old self? Or does it mean still the confused memory-losing Mom we've seen lately . . . just not having to worry about seizures anymore?"

"It's going to be okay," I said as I walked in slowly from the bathroom.

If Brint believed this, his face didn't show it. This person in front of him was far from the mom he knew. We used to talk and laugh and watch ball games together. Now, my attention was limited and my interest in anything, dwindling. Would all of my family have to get used to this new woman in their lives?

Hunter handed Brint a couple of twenties and sent him out for pizza. Our son would need some time to digest this latest news. I knew he would struggle with it. If nothing else, I knew he would feel guilt. Ever since Hunter and I made the decision our son had to go to a branch campus of Penn State to save money, rather than the main campus at University Park, we felt his animosity. He didn't want to commute—he wanted to live away from home. Most days he still had a chip on his shoulder. I hated to add on anything more.

No sooner had Brint started down the driveway than I saw Ann pull up. She had a huge smile on her face. Her field trip must have gone well. I cringed at the thought of bringing her down. She had been so full of optimism after my appointment with Dr. Kifer. This news was going to be hard to hear. Everything was going perfectly in her life—except for me.

"What's going on here? Did something happen?"

I wanted to answer her, but my mouth wouldn't move.

"Your mom had an incident today at work. She's okay but she's a little worn out."

"What happened?" Ann asked again. "Did you fall or . . .."

"I had a seizure," I said, cursing the words as they left my mouth. "But I'm perfectly fine now."

Ann wrapped her arms around me in a huge hug. I could feel her trembling.

"We called Dr. Kifer and he is putting me on a new drug. Maybe that Topamax was doing more good than we thought. I don't know what this seizure-stuff is all about, but I think this Depakote will help."

I filled her in on some of the specifics, but saw no point in adding more grief to her day. I changed the subject as soon as I could.

"So tell me about the field trip! I want to know all about it."

Ann hesitated, but agreed to move on. The sparkle in her eyes came back. She was a teacher through-and-through. She was excellent at the job already. I was so proud.

Hunter left to pick Callie up at cheerleading practice. He wanted to prepare her for what she was coming home to.

"Where's Mom?" I heard her ask as she dropped her backpack at the door. I took a breath and prepared for the second whirlwind coming.

A long hug gave Callie some peace, but talking things out would be instrumental in getting her to understand it. I made a point of staying positive, and minimizing my condition. The worst was over, according to my plan. The new medicine would work, I would get back to normal, and life would go merrily along.

"You know nothing is going to keep Mom down for long," Hunter whispered in Callie's ear.

I smiled when I heard his words. But I wasn't so sure he was right this time. Something terrifying was going on. It was more than migraines, more than hormones. Everything I did was being affected—my job, my family, my day-to-day activities. Nothing was normal anymore. 'Being clumsy' couldn't explain my falls. A 'senior moment' couldn't write-off my forgetfulness. And now a seizure? Something was terribly wrong.

I took a deep breath and tried to calm myself down. Why didn't I see this happening? How could changes this drastic be going on in my life without my noticing? Did everyone else see these things? My mind wandered to the other teachers laughing at me after school. Of course, they noticed! How could they not? It was plain to everyone but me.

I felt the panic attack sweep over me and diminish my senses. I was scared. I was horrified. Things weren't in my control anymore. The rapid breathing, the sweating—they were masters on their own. They had control now. I needed to get used to this. This was going to be my life!

I picked up my laptop and said a silent prayer for clarity. I needed to research again. I needed to find some answers. That was the only thing that was going to calm me down.

I googled fatigue, but this time I added fast heartrate. I'd suffered from my heart racing for the past few weeks. I tried to overlook it, or blame it on nervousness, but it was more than that. The two symptoms together brought up two ailments. Anemia was the first. It said, a condition in which the blood doesn't have enough healthy red blood cells. I could add to my symptoms shortness of breath if this was indeed my diagnosis. I opened the desk drawer and pulled out the results of the bloodwork Dr. Curtis had ordered. My red blood cell count was normal. I felt both relief and defeat upon seeing the news.

"I didn't want anemia, anyway," I said out loud to myself. "Move on to the second ailment!"

Anxiety Disorder stared me straight in the face. It read, a mental health disorder characterized by feelings of worry, anxiety, or fear that are strong enough to interfere with daily life. Usually self-diagnosable. Lab tests not required. Caused by stress that is out of proportion to the impact of the event, inability to set aside a worry, and restlessness. Whole body fatigue. Sweating. Cognitive lack of concentration. Racing thoughts. Unwanted thoughts. Nausea. Trembling. Irritability.

Bingo! I found a winner! This had to be it! Every symptom of mine was listed! Of course, stress! That's what I thought all along! I had myself almost giddy! I didn't need to go talk to anyone. I didn't need a doctor! I just needed to stay away from stress! I was jubilant! I was normal! I just needed to live stress-free! It sounded ridiculous, but I could do it. I loved my job, my family, my life! And the seizures...well, the seizures were being stopped by medicine. I was going to be fine. I just needed to quit worrying and enjoy life. I fell into bed, tired, but happy. Tomorrow would be better.

The sick feeling in the pit of my stomach when I woke up the next morning wouldn't go away. All I could think about was yesterday's seizure. No matter how much I tried to talk myself into a happy start for the day, it wouldn't work. Unwanted thoughts—I remembered. This was definitely an example.

"Ready to go, Mom?" Brint called from the kitchen. He was driving me to work and back today.

"Just a minute, sweetie!" I needed a minute...more than a minute. I needed time to give myself a pep talk. Just a few more days. I could do this!

I met Brint in the car.

"Thanks so much for doing this, Brint. I really appreciate you getting up early and..."

"It's not a big deal, Mom!" Brint tried to reassure me.

"I know you hate to get up early," I repeated.

"It's fine...really," he added. I knew my son—very well. He would much rather be sleeping in his bed, celebrating the semester being over than driving his mom to school. But this was a necessity. His small contribution was part of my family pulling together.

My students, after a few awkward, uncomfortable minutes, that Monday morning, realized I was the same old Mrs. Church. I was back to school and, in their world, everything was better. But, in reality, nothing was better. I truly wasn't feeling well at all. And I had so much work to do! It was becoming that every time I stood up from my desk to do something, either

I forgot what it was or I didn't have the energy to even start the task. My symptoms were increasing. I gave the credit to stress.

"Need some help?" The girl at the classroom door was like a gift from heaven.

"Not unless you're a little fairy who can twirl around this room and take down the penguins." I didn't know who she was, but I prayed she wasn't joking.

"Do you remember me, Mrs. Church? I had you for fourth grade."

"I'm sorry," I said, without making my brain strain. "I'm having a pretty hectic day and I'm afraid it would be forever till I guessed."

The girl gave me a smile. "I'm Trisha Wisconski. You always used to tease me and say 'I wonder if Miss Wisconski will ever go to Wisconsin?'"

"Of course I remember you," I lied. I couldn't remember all of the names of the students I had now. "What are you doing here now?"

"I'm a senior at the high school. I still needed some more hours of community service before the end of the school year. They told me to report to your room."

There was no point in feeling embarrassed. It had to be obvious to everyone, I needed the help

"Well, Trisha, I am so happy to see you again. I mean, I am REALLY happy to see you. One look at this room, though, and you'll want to go anyplace else."

"Not a chance," the girl said, rubbing her hands together. "You were always my favorite teacher. I want to help. Just point to what you want done."

I said a silent prayer of thanks and showed her the ladder in the corner of the room. I'd been putting off using it for weeks. In my shaky state, I was too afraid I would fall. Taking down and hanging up seemed like a rather easy request to Trisha.

By this time, the students were done with their math and were getting a little too rambunctious. I gave Trisha full reign and called the children up to the front carpet to hear me read the next chapter of 'Old Yeller'. I sank into my rocking chair and captured the students' attention with a quick summary of what happened last in the book.

By the third page, I was asleep. I awoke to the taps of little fingers on my shoulders.

"Mrs. Church, are you getting sick again like last week?" That question was enough to jostle me awake. It also made me sick to my stomach.

"You silly guys," I said, with a pasted smile on my face, "I am just teasing. I wasn't really sleeping."

Most of the children started to laugh and fired back with their cries that they knew it all along. I was just thankful they bought it.

I went to the closet and got out a stack of construction paper. "Use this paper to make anything you want," I said to the children. This was so unlike me. Usually I had projects planned out and executed with precision.

I could feel Trisha's eyes on me as I moved about the room. Did she see me sleeping a few minutes ago? Was I acting strange to her? I wanted to know but I didn't dare ask. I couldn't bear to hear the answer.

With Trisha's help, the last four days of school came and went. She stripped my room, organized the art cupboard, and collected all the books. On her last day, I slipped her two twenties and wished her good luck.

I still had some 'teacher stuff' to do, but no ambition left within me. I felt like I finished a marathon. I promised the principal I would be in some evening to finish up my work. Instead, I sent Ann and Callie out to the school with a list of tasks. I'd made it to the end of a horrendous year. I knew if I went back there when it was dark and empty, I'd relive that seizure day all over again. I just couldn't handle that right now.

All along, I had been so nervous about just doing my job at school, I didn't realize how scared I was about my health. I just thought—make it to the end of the year and you'll be fine. I was seeing, this wasn't the case. I was exhausted, mentally and physically. I spent most of the first few days at home sleeping. I allowed myself to withdraw from the world and forget about everything. My anxiety disorder, if that was indeed what it was, was in full swing.

Hunter hinted several times about me getting back in touch with the real world. He encouraged me to join in on trips to the grocery store or pharmacy. I balked at first, but knew if I didn't, he would be convinced I was sicker and make me go to the doctor. That's exactly what I needed, but the fog in my brain made it too difficult to see. I didn't know it was this obvious to others.

Every day that passed, I felt more lethargic. Sleeping was the only thing I was good at. I would have been content to stay in my bed forever. Nothing made me motivated.

"I need some things at Walmart, Mom. Want to tag along?" Ann's words were meant to sound so welcoming. I had just taken a two-hour nap and had a bit of energy.

"I'd love it!" I lied, "If you're sure I won't slow you down."

My daughter laughed at my words, but she and I both realized the reality of things. Taking me along also entailed holding on to me when I walked and helping me in and out of the car. It was no picnic for the person assisting me.

Ann pulled in to Walmart and stopped at the door. I knew this was my cue to exit. Any further into the parking lot would exhaust my energy to the point where I couldn't walk through the store. She helped me out and sat me on a bench like a little kid. I was embarrassed. But more than that, I was frustrated. I so wanted to be back to the life I had before. . .before whatever this was took me over.

Three different people came up to me and asked how I was doing. I had no idea if I knew them or if they were just trying to be friendly. I tried striking up a conversation, but my words came out garbled. That was something I hadn't experienced before. I prayed it would go away before Ann met up with me.

I stayed unusually silent as my daughter maneuvered me through the aisles. I finally asked her a question, wishing with all my heart for my words to make sense. This time they did. I wanted to sit down. I had stumbled twice while I was walking and didn't want Ann to be burdened with me as she shopped. She sat me in a chair by the pharmacy and promised to be quick.

I glanced at the medicines on the shelves and wondered, innocently, if there was something there to help me. I could sense my health worsening since school was out. Wasn't there a pill or something to make me better? My thoughts were almost childlike. I was glad when Ann returned.

My trip to the store wore me out. I fell asleep in the car, then slept for three hours after we got home. I relied on someone else to do the cooking and cleaning. I was just a bystander, watching my life go on without me. At night, Hunter and Brint would help me up the ten steps to the second floor. By this time of day, I was usually so weak that I stumbled, even with help. My falls were becoming almost commonplace. This way of life was becoming our norm.

The last straw for me came the evening my husband and I attempted a very short walk on a nearby dirt road. I had rested all day on the couch and had a little burst of energy. I wanted to get out and feel normal. It was a straight stretch, one we had walked hundreds of times before. He finally acquiesced.

I mustered up my strength as I started the trail. I vowed I wouldn't tire, or give in to stupid thoughts telling me I was weak. I managed just a tad of the trail I used to briskly tackle everyday only a year ago. Now, I could feel my body resisting the commands I was giving it to move on. Hunter said I appeared to be a little tired. This was an understatement. We turned around to head back. I couldn't walk. Every step I took was off to the right. It took

Hunter an hour to renegotiate each step of mine to get me back home. We both knew, after that, despite the rest and the positive thinking, I wasn't getting better. Whatever this was, it wasn't going away.

"Lisa, I think it's time we find a doctor. You are getting worse."

The fear in my heart when he said that came to life. As much as I wanted to be better, I didn't want to go to a doctor. When people had something serious and they weren't getting better, the doctor always confirmed bad news. I was sure I must have cancer or a brain tumor or something destroying my body.

"Please, Hunter. Just give me another few days. I want to look on the internet again."

"Honey, this isn't something Google can answer for us. We need a doctor to check you out. "

"But there has to be someone out there, feeling the way I am feeling, walking how I am walking, and deteriorating the way. . ." I couldn't finish the sentence. I said it in my head—deteriorating the way I am, sadly and suddenly. For one of the first times, I broke down in front of Hunter. Up till now, I'd done my crying alone. But this time, I didn't have a choice.

My husband handed me my laptop with a warning. "Tonight you can research your symptoms, Tomorrow, we'll talk about the doctor again."

It took me hours to do the research. My mind was foggy and I kept falling asleep. I tried to make the most of my brief moments of clarity. Tonight, I googled memory loss and balance problems. There were hundreds of things the websites wanted me to claim as my own. I went from having a chemical imbalance to an inner-ear infection to being a hypochondriac. I swore I had everything from Multiple Sclerosis to early Alzheimer's. But I finally settled on telling my family I thought I had Lyme disease. It was a little-talked-about illness introduced and spread by ticks found on deer and small rodents in Pennsylvania and several other states. Locals had treated their dogs with preventative medications for years. But it was just in the past year or so that *people* in our area appeared to be contracting it. The list of possible symptoms was a mile long, and I didn't have many of the prominent ones—no tick bite, no bull's eye rash, no joint achiness. But it was something to consider. As soon as I had a 'good' day, I would read more about this disease and learn how to fix it. I felt somewhat relieved I had an idea of what might be wrong.

Up until now, as long as the seizures were stifled, I considered myself to be getting better. But, as my husband sternly pointed out to me today, other symptoms were too prevalent now. My walking, my talking, my control of self was fading. And nothing I read on the internet was going to shine a light and magically fix me. It was time to give in and admit I truly needed medical attention. This wasn't a 'passing virus' as I so often referred to it. It was time to give it a real name and get it fixed.

Relieved at my revelation, my husband consoled me "Let's talk things over with your sisters tomorrow and see what they suggest. We'll get started on this together and get you back on track."

I let my thoughts run wild, hoping, as I always did, that the chaos in my brain would organize itself and reveal the secret. It didn't. I nodded anyway and accepted the answer. My sisters were licensed practical nurses at my doctor's office. I'd kept my increase in symptoms private up till now, mainly just to spark no concern. But now, I needed them, along with any other help I could get.

"I'm sure I'll be much better in the morning," I said confidently, unaware that I'd used that same line every night for two weeks. I closed my eyes, still wondering why I would be seeing my sisters the next day.

"I'll take Mom to Trey's birthday party if you want to just hang out at home or even go fishing." Ann's words to her dad were said in front of me. I tried to pick up on pieces of their conversation. I trembled at the thought of my incoherent thoughts. I wanted to just crawl back in bed and hide from the world that was becoming too big and confusing for me. I listened for my husband's response. I needed to get out of the house. I needed to learn who Trey was.

I could tell my husband was contemplating the option. It reminded me my condition was having an effect on everyone in the family.

"You know what?" I heard Hunter say, "I think I will take you up on that. I could use a few hours to catch up on some things around here."

Ann smiled at his answer.

"Make sure you talk to Aunt Glenda and Aunt Wanda about Mom!" Hunter's words put a concerned look on Ann's face. Was there anyone who wasn't being hurt by this?

I started stressing over what I was going to wear. I ended up trusting Ann to pick out something appropriate. My judgment was off in everything. Selecting a dress, even rummaging in the closet, was too much for me.

By noontime, I had heard enough comments from my kids about Trey to jiggle my memory. He was my brother's son. How I ever could forget that was troubling to me. I digested the comments and moved on. I had to keep up with my surroundings. It would be too easy for me to get lost in the confusion of my life.

The day was hot—almost 90 degrees. It took about an hour for Ann to drive us to Ty's. When we arrived, we joined the other family and friends in the back yard. I grabbed a few chips from the table and tried to act like a part of the gang. Maybe seeing my brothers and sisters would make me forget my troubles. Maybe my mind would revert back to the days when I was 10 years old, growing up in a lively house with my mom and four siblings.

I sat outside with another family I didn't know. Should I know them? Apparently they had a three-year-old running and playing with my nephew. I made small talk the best I could, but I could feel my resistance to the everyday world starting to sink in.

I wanted to ask one of my children to get me a cold drink. But when I saw them, talking and laughing and not worrying about me for once, I held off. This illness or condition of mine, was affecting their every move. I wanted to see the smiles on their faces and hear their laughter a little longer. Finally, Callie moved my way.

"I'm hot," I said to Callie, hoping she wouldn't pick up on my irritable mood.

"I hear there are cold drinks in the house," she said, helping me stand up. "Let's go."

I welcomed the chance to leave the yard. The noise of happy youngsters had become annoying. It was unusual for me to think like that. As a teacher of little ones, it took a lot for children to get on my nerves. Perhaps it was the high temperature today. But the thought of a cool drink in the air-conditioned house sounded more than appealing. We headed inside, ready for some lemonade with plenty of ice.

The blast of cool air in the kitchen felt overwhelming after being in that hot sun. The room was crowded. My head began to swirl. I wanted to get a drink and sit down.

"Those ribs look spectacular," I heard Brint say to my brother. It was the last thing I remember.

I hit the floor hard, landing on my side as I was starting to seize. I could sense the horror the others were feeling. I heard crying. I heard shouting. I heard the rattling of my body writhing on the kitchen tile. It seemed to last forever. Finally, I stopped moving. I opened my eyes.

I watched everyone around me. They seemed to know what to do. My sister-in-law picked up the phone. Ty moved everyone back. Wanda put me on my side. I could see a look of horror on Callie's face.

"What's wrong?" I asked her. "What happened?"

My daughter couldn't speak. It was as if she was frozen, except for the tears trickling down her cheeks.

"You had a seizure, Mom." I could see Brint's blue eyes looking into mine. Were they always this blue, I wondered.

"Brint?" I said, pronouncing his name slowly. "Can you help me?"

"The ambulance is on its way, Mom," my son replied.

"I want to sit up," I said, unclear about what was happening. I put my hand down to help myself up.

"Oh, there's something spilled here," I said, unaware I was sitting in my own urine. Ann came to my rescue. Paper towels in hand, she grabbed hold of my arm and helped me upright. She wiped my hands and the back of my legs, never letting on what would have embarrassed me tremendously. I could hear an ambulance wailing from afar, getting louder with each passing moment. Finally realizing what was going on, I shut my eyes tightly and murmured, "This wasn't supposed to happen again." I shut out the world and let the medics take me away.

It took only minutes to get to the local hospital. Ann rode with me in the ambulance while Brint stayed behind to call his dad. I could remember Callie's flustered and shocked look as they loaded me into the vehicle.

The ER doctor ran through a list of questions. It reminded me of my last seizure. Ann did most of the talking this time. She answered his questions and asked more.

By the time Hunter got there, I was vomiting into a basin. I felt physically and emotionally sick. I couldn't comprehend what was going on. I could hear talking off to the side but couldn't hone in on the words or subject matter. When Hunter finally came near me, I felt a rush of relief.

"It's going to be okay, babe. They're taking you down for a few tests just to make sure everything is good." He smiled at me. I could see he was nervous. I tried to smile back. I couldn't. I felt devoid of emotion. I lay back on the bed and waited to be taken down the hall. I shut my eyes tight. Make this all go away.

A series of tests showed nothing. Everything appeared normal. That was good news. But better news would have explained what was wrong. How could I go from standing one minute, to being sprawled on the floor in a puddle of pee the next?

A group of people entered the room. Callie stood out to me most. I gave her an extra long hug. "I'm going to be fine, Sweetie."

"But that was a seizure, Mom! You said no more seizures. And you had one. I saw you! It was horrible!"

My heart ached. I kept causing pain.

I pulled her down beside me on the bed. My appearance did nothing to soothe her. I looked hot and tired and totally exhausted. My clothes had been changed from the classy white sundress I had on earlier to a hospital gown. I smelled like sweat and pee.

"The doctor said he had one more thing to check and then I could go." I tried to sound optimistic.

My mom and Brint appeared next in my room. A few leftover tears wet my face. I stood up slowly to greet them.

"I'm okay, Mom, really," I said, starting to cry all over again. She hugged me. I hugged Brint next. Why was he so white? He looked to me for good news. What should I say? Hunter's entrance into our inner-circle was welcome.

"The doctor here just got off the phone with Dr. Kifer. He feels the drug he put you on a few weeks ago, this Depakote, hasn't taken full effect. It's not built up in your system yet. That's why you had the seizure. He said to give the medicine another day or two to reach full-strength, and you should be done with seizures."

"That makes sense," my relieved mother said, reflecting back on her 40-plus years of service as a registered nurse.

"I agree," Brint chimed in.

I heard the words but didn't find the relief the other listeners had. Okay, no more seizures. But what about my mixed-up speech, my falls, my reasoning? Yes, I added a new one to my list of symptoms—reasoning. I'd been denying problems here, or should I say ignoring them.

In actuality, I had given up over the last months on offering opinions or questioning things. I avoided group conversations because I couldn't follow along. I couldn't collect my thoughts fast enough to keep up. Instead, I learned to keep quiet—agree with what was being said. I was afraid of embarrassing myself. This problem with reasoning was real. Hiding my insecurities from everyone was a new task tagged on to my never-ending list of woes. My life was a mess.

My husband put a towel over the passenger seat for the car ride home. My dress was still wet from my incontinence when I seized earlier. I put my head back on the seat and closed my eyes. I was spent. I just wanted to curl up in a ball and be left alone.

The next two weeks I slept. Without the challenges of school to deal with, I permitted myself to indulge in catnaps as often as I wanted. I was either in the sun on a lounge chair or, in the evening, I took sanctuary in my bedroom. I turned on the ceiling fan to drown out the noise of the real world. The hum of the blades always calmed me.

At least during those times, I was masking the other problems that plagued me. All of my previous symptoms continued at heightened levels. I couldn't walk. Without a person at my side, I would run into things or fall or do both. I had so many bruises on me that I looked like a battered wife. I had fractured a rib when I fell at my brother's, making everything, even breathing, painful. My thinking was getting cloudy, or should I say cloudier, than ever before. I was gaining more weight, and yet, I wasn't eating. I should have been scared, but I didn't have the faculties to recognize it.

"We're calling Dr. Kifer for an appointment," Hunter announced to Ann and me one morning. "I want him to see you."

I gave my husband a blank stare. He could have told me he was calling the surgeon general and I wouldn't have reacted any differently. My desire to fight was collapsing.

I eavesdropped on the phone conversation as I stretched out on the couch. I wouldn't be able to put my thoughts together to handle the phone call on my own. I cringed as Hunter went over my list of symptoms: exhaustion, unsteadiness, trembling, trouble with words, foggy memory, weight gain, two seizures. Hunter stopped talking and concentrated on what the nurse on the other end of the line was saying. There was a long silence, then I heard him pleading.

"I know what the doctor said, but Lisa really needs to be seen! I know you don't treat seizures, but Dr. Kifer knows her history and the medications she takes. He prescribed the seizure medicine she is on. If he could just see her, maybe he could figure out what's wrong."

Hunter was not giving up. "Can't you talk to him again? He put her on Depakote after her first seizure and told the ER doctor to have her see him if she didn't get better."

There was another long pause. Hunter sighed and put the phone on speaker. The receptionist continued.

"Dr. Kifer says your wife is just stressed because of the seizures. He doesn't want to see her in his office right now. He said to tell her to get plenty of exercise, drink lots of water, and perhaps we may want to set her up an appointment with a psychiatrist."

"For what?" Hunter yelled into the phone.

"She may be imagining things," the receptionist politely responded. "She may just be nervous waiting for the full dose of Depakote to take effect. Do you want me to set up an appointment for her at the psychiatrist? This is the middle of June. The psychiatrist doesn't have any openings until mid-August."

"We don't want to see a psychiatrist!" Hunter pleaded. "We want an appointment with the neurologist!"

"He doesn't want to see her at this time."

The words fell on deaf ears. Even Ann's entreaties in the background didn't change the receptionist's mind. My husband hung up, shaking his head.

"I don't believe it!" I heard Ann say. "He won't see her?"

"He thinks she is just nervous about the past seizures and the new medicine she is on. He said she is suffering from anxiety and a wild imagination."

"You can't imagine a seizure!" Ann interjected.

"I know," my husband said, rubbing his temple. "He wants her to see a psychiatrist in August."

"I heard." Ann paused to collect her thoughts. "Dad," Ann added, forgetting I was within earshot, "she could be dead by then." My daughter threw herself into her dad's shoulder, burying her face to hide the tears and sobs. She was trembling. I was oblivious to how serious the situation was.

The conversation between the two of them was one of sadness and despair. They didn't know what to do. This doctor had been the man we had always trusted! And now, all of a sudden, he was just going to wash his hands of us? It didn't make any sense! Had I had my wits about myself, I would have been crushed at his dismissal to such an urgent cry for help. Maybe there were no true heroes.

I grew weaker by the day, limiting my walking and tasks. I would sleep for hours upon end, and still wake up tired and confused. My memory and word retrieval issues had become so prevalent it was difficult to understand anything I said. I couldn't bathe or shower without help. My tremors worsened. I couldn't even brush my teeth on my own. Such a simple routine . . .an action toddlers learn to do, was no longer something I could manage.

One of the family members had to be assigned to me at all times to prevent me from harm. It reminded me of watching a two-year-old. What little I was able to do had to be monitored, and not everything I did made sense.

Since my neurologist had basically written me off, my husband decided a visit to our family doctor would be the next logical step. Even if Dr. Davidson couldn't diagnose me, maybe he would have some insight into where to go from here.

Dr. Davidson was already aware of most of my problems. With my sisters working in his office, they riddled him continually about my bizarre symptoms. I trusted he would be able to help. I'd seen him over the years for different things, but mainly I relied on his back and neck manipulations. Somehow he had just the right touch when it came to my spine and herniated discs. I knew he wouldn't turn us away.

"I hope you can help us, doctor," Hunter said nervously. "We aren't really sure where else to turn."

"I'm happy to do what I can," Dr. Davidson said, watching me as I tried to walk down the hall in front of him.

"We thought, at first, Lisa was just overworked. Then the seizures made us think this has to be some sort of disorder. But things have progressed quickly, and are getting much worse." Hunter's words grabbed the attention of the man. He turned toward me.

The doctor's eyes locked with mine when he saw me. I could feel his sympathy. The change in me since my last visit three months ago was staggering. The weight gain, alone, was blatantly obvious to him. My flat demeanor and passive personality were very much out of character, as he noted out loud. When he asked me to step up on the exam table, he had no idea my actions would be so pathetic. The woman who used to work out daily and take five-mile hikes was now reduced to a silhouette of who she used to be. My failed attempt to even get my leg close to the step brought tears to my eyes. I crumpled to the floor, spent and embarrassed in my defeat.

Hunter sat down on the floor right beside me and took my hand. Our worried looks were no surprise.

"She has no energy. She just wants to sleep," Hunter said. "And she's had balance problems and trouble with her speech. She is just having so many symptoms.

"First," Dr. Davidson said. "I'm very sorry this is happening to her. There is obviously something very wrong. But I'm a family doctor from the country. I don't see symptoms like this every day. Lisa needs to go to a university hospital where they have the equipment and doctors needed to figure this out."

Hunter nodded, happy at least he had gotten through to the man.

"I believe it is very important Lisa be given a PET scan. This test, also known as a Positron Emission Tomography, is a type of imaging test. It uses a radioactive substance called a tracer to look for diseases in the body. A PET scan shows how organs and tissues are working. Unfortunately, these machines are only used in very large hospitals.

"I think once Lisa gets the scan, she can be examined extensively and get an expert opinion." He scribbled down a hospital name on a card along with the name of a doctor. "I can set things up for you." His choice appeared to please my husband.

"That's great," Hunter said, elated at the prospect of more help. "My dad lives near there, so we can spend the night at his place before the exam." Ann seemed just as relieved. A large hospital, specialists. . .this would be a good thing. My appointment was made for July 5. Today was the third.

"Tomorrow we travel," Hunter said, not knowing whether I would be able to comprehend his statement. I just stared at him. It didn't make any difference to me. I was beginning to become oblivious to all the things around me. It just didn't matter. Nothing did.

❖❖❖

"Do you really want to travel five hours in the car then sit all day at a hospital while they run tests on Mom?" Hunter's words left Callie untouched.

"Dad, I want to go," Callie retorted, her voice tinged with angry denial. "I saw Mom have a seizure right before my eyes. I have helped her move around the house. I do everything I can to make things easier for her. I think I have earned the right to go!"

"There's no discussion here," he murmured. "You will be staying with Aunt Wanda."

Callie glared at him, "This is ridiculous!" she finally said. "You're treating me like a baby!"

I listened for an angry answer from Hunter. None came. All I could hear were Callie's words echoing in the silence. As much as I wished, no words would surface. I was viewing my baby learn she would be separated from her sick mother. I shuddered. As disjointed as I was, I could still sense her pain.

Hunter looked at me. He must have seen my fear. "She'll be all right," he said to me. "Tomorrow is the Fourth of July picnic out there. Callie will be much better off around family than cramped in a car for five hours."

I tried to digest what he was saying. Were we going to a picnic? And why wasn't he letting Callie come along to it? She would be good. She is little but she is old enough to behave.

"I'll have Brint take her out there in the morning. He can eat and come back home to take care of things here. The dogs will need to be let out."

I listened to my husband ramble on, making lame excuses for his actions. I was not able to realize the private hell he was going through.

Our car eased out of the driveway around noon. I had issued my tearful goodbyes to Callie and Brint earlier. I wasn't fully aware of what I was doing. I was lucid enough, though, to know I was leaving two of my babies behind.

The first portion of the five-hour-drive was uneventful. The radio played. Hunter and Ann made small talk. Intermittently, I would close my eyes and fall asleep.

"I have to pee!" I announced after three hours in the car. Hunter's face showed disappointment. I was sure he was hoping we could make it there with no diversions. He glanced over at me. I had one hand between my legs and the other on the door handle.

"I have to pee right now!" I announced, giving the door handle one firm tug. My door took wing. We were going 65 mph on the interstate and I decided to get out!

Hunter reached across the seat and grabbed my shirt. Ann cried out in the backseat and grabbed my hair. It was the only thing she could reach. Hunter slammed on his brakes and veered our car onto the berm.

"Lisa!" he shouted angrily. "What are you doing?" I didn't know it at the time, but he was terrified. His shriek was out of fear and frustration. I looked at him like he was the devil himself.

"I told you I had to pee!" I said vehemently. "Where is the bathroom?"

Hunter gave a sigh of relief, mixed with irritability and ire. He looked to Ann in the back for a little assistance.

"We have to go a little further to get to the bathroom," she said, trusting I would accept her answer.

"Well . . . okay then," I said, already forgetting I had flung my car door open. "Let me know when we get there."

I put my head back on the seat, closed my eyes, and barred the happenings of the last few moments from my mind. I felt the car pull out and heard a distant conversation. There's nothing like a summer drive, I thought. My lips curled into a smile. I nestled further into the leather seat, dreaming about a sandy beach along a tranquil, blue ocean.

"We're here," Hunter stated, giving my arm a little squeeze.

"The beach?" I said agreeably, not yet opening my eyes.

"Sorry dear, but we are at the rest stop. Remember, you needed to go to the bathroom?" I'm sure he wished he would have let the sleeping dog in me lie.

I opened my eyes abruptly, trying to transfer my thoughts from the ocean scene in my head to the brick rest-stop building.

"Where are we?" I asked, rubbing my eyes in bewilderment. "I thought we were going swimming?" I was not embarrassed. I said and did whatever I pleased lately.

"Come on, Mom," Ann smiled in the window at me. "Let's go to the bathroom."

I gave her a smile back and fumbled for the door handle. Ann opened the door herself. She held out her arm, signaling she was ready for a walk. I swiveled in my seat, facing my daughter, preparing to put my life in her hands. Hunter appeared from around the other side. I gave them each an arm and relied on their assistance to reach the entrance. I must have looked like some drunk being carried in. They were all but dragging me. Hunter looked to Ann when we entered the building successfully.

"We'll be great," Ann assured him, taking full control of me now. "Go get some coffee. We'll meet you at the car."

My husband hesitated only a second. There was little else he could do.

"Help me out here, Mom. Walk with me," Ann said softly. I wasn't really sure of what she meant, but I did realize she was the sole individual giving me aid. I stood up a little straighter and decided to oblige. We made it to the first empty stall without any ramifications.

Ann swung the door open and helped me into the close quarters.

"Get out!" I commanded, paying no mind to my daughter's feelings.

"I've got to help you, Mom," she said, trying to maneuver me front ways inside the tiny cubicle.

"I am alright, now get out!" I said, talking to her in a way I never had before. "I want you to get out."

Ann squeezed past me and exited the stall, silently. I somehow found the dexterity to lock the door.

"Finally," I said, trying to remember who just put me into this little room.

"I'm going to be right here beside you." The voice sounded like Ann's but I was certain some strange lady had taken over her body. My daughter would never lock me in a place like this.

I gave the door a slight push and realized I wouldn't be getting out of here on my own. I looked around at the small box she had put me in. When I saw the toilet, it immediately reminded me I had to go.

I could hear 'the lady' beside me unsnap her shorts and pull them down. I could picture the action. I fumbled with my own shorts and pulled them down. I flopped myself onto the seat behind me, not expecting to feel the cold plastic. I jumped in surprise, losing my balance.

"Ouch!" I squealed instantly.

"What's wrong?" the girl beside me asked. "Mom, are you okay?"

"I . . . I fell on the floor," I called out, exasperated. "I can't get up!"

The gasp on the other side of the metal wall startled me. I curled myself into a tight ball, alarmed of what would happen next.

"Are you sure you can't get up, Mom?" Ann's voice was shrouded in panic.

"No, I can't get up or I would be up!" I said in a nasty tone. I could hear the hopelessness in her voice.

"Just stay where you are," she said, up and out of her own stall now. "I am going to try to get in!"

I could hear a person jimmying the door. Was that my daughter trying to get in, or was it that mean lady who locked me in here in the first place? Was she trying to break in?

Next, I could sense someone or something trying to get near me from underneath the door.

"Get out!" I screamed, kicking my legs at the person. "Get out!"

I heard my daughter's cry.

"Is she hurting you too?" I whispered, frantically wondering how I would help her.

There was no answer. My daughter was probably injured, the latest victim of that strange woman!

I glanced down at the floor. My fall had wedged me between the toilet and the wall behind it. In my unclear state of mind, I curled myself up further, thinking it would be beneficial. Instead, it made things worse.

I could hear the rustling of someone, again crawling under the stall's door. My legs were too far away from the intruder to hurt her this time. I kicked anyway, thinking maybe I could shoo her away with good intentions.

"No! Don't come in!" I started to tremble with terror. My thoughts were racing.

I heard the lock on the door click. The person had gotten in! I mentally gave myself a pep talk, wildly trying to get further behind the toilet.

"I'm going to slide you," the girl said, attempting to pull me out.

I didn't answer. I had used up most of my energy by now. I gave in, and allowed her to pull on my legs.

"Are you hurt?" the voice asked.

"No," I said. "I'm stuck!" The forcefulness in my own voice was gone now. Somewhere I changed my mind set. I no longer cared who the person was. I just wanted off the floor.

When I got turned around, I was amazed that Ann was the one grasping my legs.

"Thank goodness you're here!" I breathed. "I couldn't find you!"

"Mom, it's going to be okay. Just let me get your legs un-wedged here." Ann straightened me out, then helped me sit up. Grappling with all of her might, she finally pulled me up to a standing position. The sigh she let out was laced with relief. I felt the same way.

"Do you still have to pee?" my daughter asked, not really sure of where to turn next.

"I never had to pee in the first place," I answered sarcastically. "I don't know why you brought me into this dump!" Again, words and a tone even I didn't recognize.

Ann pulled up my underwear and shorts, then got me out of the stall and over to the sink somehow. I'm sure she wished she could run me through a shower. The germs from that bathroom stall had to be having a field day on my body. Simply washing my hands, though, would have to do. Unfortunately for both of us, it was a press-down faucet that sprayed out a limited amount of water. My reaction time was so poor I couldn't get my hands into the water before it shut off. My daughter finally wet a paper towel and squeezed a dollop of soap from the dispenser. She washed my hands like she would a tiny child's, going in between my fingers and over the back. She got another wet one to wipe the soap off.

By the time she was done, I had gained some energy. I cradled Ann's arm in mine, and I was able to control some of my own weight. We headed gingerly toward the parking lot. I saw Hunter standing at the car. Hmm-mmm . . . I wonder what he was doing here? I gave him a kiss on the cheek as he eased me into the car.

Ann and her dad were discussing something. I thought about listening in, but I was too tired. I leaned back on the seat and shut my eyes, glad to finally have a chance to relax. Keeping up with that girl was draining!

I am sure me sleeping was the best my traveling companions could hope for at this time. They recharged when I rested. I was a baby taking a nap. As long as the little one stays asleep, you can get all kinds of things accomplished. These two, though, were trying to reach Ohio before I got awake, not do a load of laundry or put a roast in the oven.

I jostled myself back to reality after a perplexing dream. I tried to tell Hunter about it. I dreamed I got out of the car with Ann. We visited a place and played on the floor. My shoulder hurt from whatever game we were playing. I was just too tired to talk about it. I put my head back. Sleep came again.

My sleep didn't last. Minutes later, I was staring out the window. I wasn't alert. I didn't try to speak. I was more despondent than usual.

It was then I became aware of feeling hot and agitated. Within seconds, I was seizing in the front seat of the car. Our vehicle was speeding 65 mph down the interstate. Hunter was trying to find a pull-off and Ann was talking to me frantically from the backseat. My movements were incontrollable.

I was done with my episode before Hunter had a chance to pull the car off the road. Seizure number 3. I had no memory of it. I was strangely tired, but I was also feeling more like myself. I put my head back again and tried to close my eyes. Instead, I watched the city whirring past me. I must be on vacation, I thought. Visiting the city would be wonderful!

Hunter's dad and his wife, Denise, greeted us in the driveway. We had made it! I didn't know they'd be on this vacation! I stayed in the car until everyone was ready to go inside. I tried to be happy like them. But my smile wouldn't come. I needed a nap.

I sat catatonic-like on the couch through the evening. I let the world breeze on around me—trying from the inside out not to ruin the lives of the people I loved. I didn't know what was happening or why, but I did know the mood was dark and the conversations were about me. I couldn't wait for it to stop. It was starting to become scary.

My sleep was fitful. I remember Hunter holding me several times through the night, trying to calm my growing fear. Would I have to stay overnight there? Where is *there*? Random thoughts bumped around haphazardly in my brain, making me edgy and uptight. And yet, when I woke up in the morning, I felt fresh and relaxed and ready to take on a new day, even if it was just in my own fantasy world.

Ann had to take charge of dressing me. My balance was so off, my daughter had to stretch me out on the bed to pull my shorts up. I looked at her helplessly when my arms went, everywhere but in the armholes, as she was trying to put on my top. My judgment was off several inches with each try.

"We're all set!" I heard Hunter say in a perky tone.

"What time is the appointment again?" Denise asked.

Appointment? I had forgotten that was the mission of this visit. I could feel the fear growing inside me again. I didn't want to go to any appointment. I wanted to visit the city.

"8:15," Hunter answered as he took my hand. I moved it quickly so he couldn't get a grasp. I decided I wasn't going along. They could go to this appointment without me.

"Lisa, you need to get in Denise's car. It's time for us to go. We don't want to be late."

I didn't move.

"Remember you've been having trouble walking? This doctor is going to fix that all up for you." Hunter's words were not soothing. I wanted to be left alone.

"Hey," Denise interjected. "Let's go out for breakfast instead of this appointment! How's that sound, Lisa?"

Breakfast? I was hungry. Breakfast made sense. It didn't fill me with fear like that appointment.

Hunter maneuvered me into the backseat of Denise's white Nissan. It was cool and welcoming. I could sit comfortably and look out of the window on our way to the restaurant. Denise got in the driver's side and Hunter slid into the passenger's seat. Hunter's dad, Bob, and Ann were following right behind us.

My mind had grown foggier in the hour I'd been awake. I was curious about where we were and what we were doing, but not enough to verbalize it. I had a slight headache. I leaned back into the seat hoping this was going to be a very long ride. I could relax and be by myself.

The seizure came out of nowhere, just as the others had. We were speeding down the highway and, once again, I decide to have a medical crisis.

"Oh, shit!" I heard Hunter say in a faraway voice. "She's having another seizure." He spun himself around from the front seat and watched as I wriggled and flopped in the corner of the backseat. I could feel spit spraying out of my mouth. Despite my eyes rolling back in my head, I could see the terror in Hunter's eyes. He appeared very far away from me. I tried to reach for him but my arms wouldn't respond.

"I knew I should have sat back there!" he lamented, angry at himself.

Denise shook off his comment. "Should I try to pull over?" We were on the far left lane of the highway, with two crowded lanes to our right.

"No, keep driving! Keep driving!" Hunter yelled. "We need to get to the hospital now!"

By this time, I was out of the seizure. My limbs had stopped swatting and beads of sweat were trickling down my face.

"Are you okay, babe?" I heard Hunter say. I looked at him like it was just a mundane question. I nodded my head without saying a word.

The ride took another 10 minutes. I was curled up, spent and confused. I could hear my husband's voice in the distance. "This isn't supposed to be happening!" he said, shaking his head. I had heard that before. We passed the main turn for the doctor's office building and headed straight for the ER. When we reached the entrance, Denise double-parked and ran in through the double doors. She was back in a flash with a wheelchair. Hunter and Denise maneuvered me from the car to the chair. I wasn't helpful. I kept insisting on walking. Someone stepped behind the wheelchair. Was it Hunter? Was it a stranger? I could feel my anxiety growing. Where were they taking me? The person in charge put one hand on the back of my shirt to push me down so I was sitting. He gripped the wheelchair with the other. I was in a race. To where, I didn't know.

When we got inside, I could hear Hunter cascading over the usual list of symptoms with the nurse. It grew every time I heard it—seizures, balance and walking abnormalities, falling, needs help to walk, word-finding difficulties, worsening memory loss, tremors, decreased facial expression, and the latest problem—loss of peripheral vision. The list startled me. Those things can't all be about me! They must be talking about Ann! My poor sweet daughter was sick! Why didn't anyone tell me? Is that why we were at this place? Was it a hospital?

I tugged on Hunter's shirt sleeve. "Why can't she see?" I asked. "Why can't she see?" The words didn't faze him. As long as I wasn't rolling around on the floor peeing myself, I was invisible. I could feel a deep anger stirring inside me.

"She's had two seizures in the last 24 hours," I heard Denise say to the woman. I wanted to be heard! I was getting madder. I wanted to yell at the world! But just then, before I could open my mouth, I wet myself and threw up. Another seizure. Why couldn't anyone make it stop?

The doctor on staff in the ER did a brief exam and admitted me right away. A nurse handed a drab gray gown to Ann and asked her to change me. Without too much fuss, I was promoted from a visitor to a patient.

I was sent to neurology and seen by a doctor, but I was unable to pay any attention to him or his examination.

"Let's get an EEG today," I thought I heard him say.

The doctor's words seemed to impress everyone but me. Hunter and Denise were hanging on his every word. Ann, on the other hand, was standing beside me, rubbing my arm gently. I heard, as if from a distance, the doctor say he would go over the chart Dr. Davidson faxed. The others nodded their understanding and stepped back. The doctor left the room hurriedly, as if to remind everyone he was busy and I was just a blip on the screen.

A young man with Batman scrubs pushed the EEG machine into the room. I was wired up, and had heard I was to remain wired up, until 5:30 a.m. tomorrow. I was too exhausted to fight.

The day was taxing for everyone. I slept through most of it, awakening now and then crying to go home. Ann and Hunter kept giving me excuses and matter-of-fact answers. I became combative with the nurses. Ann was the best at keeping me calm, so it seemed the nurses on duty found her a welcome addition to the fold. She spent the night dozing on and off in the orange vinyl chair near my bed.

"Ouch, that hurts!" I cried early the next morning, as the technician in a pink outfit started to strip me of the wires. She began the routine of unpeeling the electrodes stuck to my head.

"You're pulling out my hair!" I shouted, mistaking the wires for sections of my hair. I prayed I wouldn't be bald by the end of her task. Did my looks really matter? I was just going to die anyway. Nobody knew what I had and I was getting worse. I almost felt dead already. I pictured myself in a wooden box, hairless and dressed in a Batman gown. I screamed some more.

"So sorry," the nurse said, without skipping a beat. She finished and left the room. I scanned my surroundings, trying to figure out where I was. No family, no friends . . . this looked like a hospital. But I had learned I couldn't trust my judgment. Just because I think I'm in a hospital doesn't mean I am. My mind wandered, trying to piece together how I got here. A car wreck?

A fall? I leaned back on the pillow and shut my eyes. Blocking out ideas was easier than trying to figure them out.

I must have fallen asleep for a short time. When I next opened my eyes, I was surprised to see Ann. She smiled brightly and said, "Good morning." I smiled back but couldn't find my words.

"Dad is trying to find the doctor so we can get the results of the test."

I just stared blankly at her. What test? A school test? Why wasn't I in my classroom? I wanted to interrogate Ann, but Hunter and a woman I didn't know walked in before I could start.

"Hi, Mrs. Church, my name is Dr. Gates. How are you today?"

When I didn't answer right away, she started the conversation without me.

"So, the neurologist examined you yesterday in the ER. Let's see, his notes say: 'Exam shows mild language and memory impairment, marked truncal ataxia without a significant appendicular dysmetria, some motor perseveration, heel-shin apraxia (mild). Findings point to a progressive cortical disorder. Recurrence of old or new onset of different seizure disorder. Consider CJD, paraneoplastic, other CNS inflammatory or infiltrative meningeal disorder.'"

I could see Ann typing words into her phone. What was she writing? Why couldn't I see? Why couldn't I write too?

"As for the EEG test," the doctor continued, "It showed mild to moderate diffuse encephalopathy. No epileptiform discharge or EEG seizures were recorded. Exam at time of admission was noted for mild language and memory impairment, marked truncal ataxia and some motor perseveration."

Who was she talking to? Was she speaking in another language?

"What is truncal ataxia?" I heard Hunter ask. I was impressed. He sounded smart.

"Truncal ataxia is often known as drunken sailor's gait or staggering."

Hunter nodded and let the woman finish her reading. "Family said the patient's one-year history showed rapid progressive worsening of gait disturbance, memory loss, tremors, aphasia, and peripheral vision disturbances."

Finally, I thought! Someone figured out my eye trouble! I'd been trying to describe it to Hunter for weeks but didn't know how to explain it. I felt like I was in a tunnel. Why couldn't I have just told Hunter that? He would have understood. He is smart. Or was he a drunk? He was a sailor in the Navy. My mind was blurry again. I hoped I wasn't going to have another seizure.

"So, what does this mean, doctor?" I heard Ann ask.

"Well, it means we're not sure what is causing her problems," the doctor said in her icy monotone. "I doubled the milligrams of Depakote that she was on to 500 milligrams twice a day. Hopefully that will take care of the seizures."

I could see Ann squirming, but I wasn't sure why.

"My mom is very sensitive to some drugs," my daughter said rather meekly. "I don't know if you should double this medicine so quickly."

The doctor looked at Ann with a smirk. "And where did you get your medical degree, honey? I think I know what I'm doing."

Was she being mean to Ann? Why did she smile like that?

Hunter glanced at Ann, then turned his attention toward me. He whispered that this doctor was going to make me better. I had to believe that.

It was then, without anyone knowing, I felt a calm sense of relief wash over my body. Although I appeared out of touch, I could still feel some semblance of reality within my soul. My brain was working like it should. This *is* a good place for me to be! You can't get a better hospital! They're topnotch! They'll find out what's wrong and fix me up! Hunter said they would! There's nothing to be frightened about! I was rambling inside my own head. I tried to get my thoughts out, but my brain couldn't connect with my mouth. Oh, where was my mom? She would know what to do!

"I'm going to order some tests," Dr. Gates announced. "We'll know more after those results come back."

Everyone seemed to relax. The doctor left the room. I could hear words like encephalopathy, gait disturbance, aphasia tossed back and forth between my husband and daughter. I wanted to ask them what they thought, but I had to shut my eyes and lean back against my pillow. The white blur of the walls was making me dizzy.

A needle piercing my arm brought my faculties back for the moment. "Ouch!" I squealed. "You're hurting me!" I tried to pull my arm back, but the woman in blue pajamas had a tight grasp on me.

"We'll be done here in a minute, honey. Keep still." The woman's words infiltrated my brain, jumbling with the random thoughts from earlier. Her good mood and pleasant words were as piercing to my head as the needle sticking in my arm. I felt sick.

"I think I might throw up on you," I uttered. The woman kept right on going, filling one vial up after another.

"Wouldn't be the first time," the lady responded with no worry. Her hold on me grew tighter. I winced at her touch.

"Let me go!" I demanded. "You're being mean!" Nothing changed. The tug and pull—the rhythm of the vials being filled—I believed she was enjoying it.

"I want you to stop!" I said again louder. I tried to pull my arm back, but I hadn't the strength. Her tight grasp kept me under control.

It seemed like forever but she finally released me. My wheelchair took flight again. I shut my eyes and put my head back. I felt the breeze as someone wheeled me quickly back to where we had started.

I felt strange right away. I think she left the needle in my arm! It was pounding and pulsating. Did she take out all of my blood? My thoughts were frightening and scattered.

I was so relieved to see my husband and daughter enter the room! "They hurt me!" I shrieked, trying to stand up. "The lady tried to shake all my blood out!" I could see concern on their faces, but why weren't they strategizing? They needed to protect me!

The lady who had taken me to get my blood drawn helped my husband situate me back in bed. I thought I could do it myself. I wanted to do it myself, but they wouldn't allow it. I made myself stiff and straight. I would show *them* who's in charge of me.

"Please, Lisa," my husband blurted. "You need to get back in this bed."

"She didn't even put a BAND-AID on me! She poked holes in me! What if all my blood drains out?"

Reluctantly, I allowed them to pull me from the wheelchair and plunk me into bed. I crossed my arms in defiance.

"I will be right back," the lady said matter-of-factly. "We're going to hook up an EEG. I just need to get the machine."

"Machine?" I questioned out loud. Ann ignored my remark and smoothed out the sheets on my bed. She fluffed up my pillow and sat down on the edge.

"You're doing great, Mom," she said.

Great at what? Sitting in a chair? Getting in bed?

I tried to smile at my daughter. Her words were confusing to me, yet soothing. I put my head back on my pillow. I was too tired to give her a rough time. I was missing my habit of taking several naps throughout the day. I would welcome one now, if given a chance.

When the nurse returned, I slept soundly as she connected the electrodes to my head again. When I next awoke, several hours had passed.

I was served a supper of vegetable soup and a toasted cheese sandwich. My daughter did her best to feed me, but I followed through on only a bite or two. I kept trying to give the rest away to Ann and Hunter. They promised me they would have their supper soon. It didn't change my mind.

By 6:30 p.m., I realized there were wires pasted to my head. I tried to pull them out. A nurse was called in several times before I gave up on my mission to free myself of these restraints.

"I'm ready to go home," I said to my husband. "When is my appointment over?"

"Soon, babe, I promise. We just need to stay long enough for them to find out what's wrong. Then we'll go home." He squeezed my hand. I wanted to cry.

"Mom, how are you?" I heard Callie's anxious voice on the other end of the phone.

"Hi, Sweetie. How are you doing?" I was having a minute of sanity. The phone call from Callie was meant to calm the nerves of each of us. Ann had arranged it.

"I miss you," I could hear the sadness in her voice.

"I miss you too," I said.

My oldest daughter seemed satisfied the conversation could go on without her presence. She gave me a smile and stepped out of the room. I continued on with my talk.

"Are you being good? You know I will give you stickers if you are."

"Yes, Mom," Callie giggled.

I could picture her chatting on the phone and laughing. She was so little! I couldn't remember if she was three or four.

"Is the babysitter treating you nice?"

"Mom, stop joking. I haven't had a babysitter in years. You know I'm at Leah's."

I let the words sink in. My little sweetie must be mixed up.

"How did you get to Leah's?" I asked.

"Brint brought me," she said, sounding a little concerned at my words.

"Don't tell me he took you all the way there on his bike!" My voice was full of alarm. I couldn't imagine a 25-mile bike ride with Callie on the back.

"Mom, you're scaring me."

"Where is Leah's mother?" I asked, becoming more and more agitated.

"She's not here."

"What?" I could feel the anger building inside of me again.

"Callie, you get your stuff together. I'm coming to pick you up."

"You're coming home now? Really?"

"Yes, really," I answered tersely.

"You stay put and no more long bike rides!"

"Okay, Mom. I love you!"

The words touched my heart as they always did when one of my children said them to me.

"I love you too." My sentiment was genuine, but my words were laced with anger. Why did we ever leave Brint and Callie alone? They are too young!

I dropped Ann's phone down on the bed and stared at it. That's a nice shade of blue, I thought. Did it match the sky?

Ann entered the room to the perplexed look on my face.

"How is everything with Callie?" she asked.

"How would I know?" I answered in a rather bothered tone.

"You were talking to her on the phone when I got called out of the room."

"Who called you out of the room? What did they want? You shouldn't be talking to strangers, you know."

Ann's look of disappointment at my behavior change from just a few minutes ago went unnoticed by me. I was in the mood to scold. I gave it to Callie, now I would give it to her.

"It's okay, Mom. I didn't talk to anyone but the doctor. Remember that nice lady who talked to us yesterday?"

"There are no nice people here. Now we need to get going. I need to pick Wanda up."

My gift of coherency was short-lived. My words weren't making sense, even inside my head.

"Wanda?" Ann repeated.

"Yes, she needs a ride. She can't be trusted to be out on her own."

Ann stared at me for a few seconds before answering.

"Mom, Wanda doesn't need a ride. She's at home. We will see her in a few days."

"No, I just told her to stay there. I'm picking her up."

My adrenaline rush edged me to the side of the bed before Ann could react. My legs hadn't supported me in days. I crumbled to the floor.

"Mom!" my daughter cried. She was down on the floor beside me within seconds.

"Are you hurt?" she asked, helping me to sit up.

"Why would I be hurt?" I snapped.

"You fell from your bed," Ann said, still giving me the once-over.

"This is stupid!" I shouted. "Why am I even in bed? It is not dark out!"

A nurse rushed into my room. Did she hear me fall? Did she hear me yell? Maybe *she* knows why I'm in bed!

If I expected her to be my friend, I was wrong. She grabbed me under my arms and pulled me backwards. Ann helped her hoist me up and onto the bed. They swung my legs around and kept hold of me in case I wanted a do-over.

"Mrs. Church, you can't get out of bed. Your legs are a little too weak right now to hold you."

"Then fix them!" I demanded. "I have to go pick up Wanda."

Ann stepped in front of the nurse. Perhaps if I didn't see the woman, I would be a little easier to deal with.

"Mom, we'll get Wanda in a little bit. I will call her and tell her we'll be a little late."

My daughter's words satisfied me for the moment.

"As long as she knows we're coming," I said, relaxing just a tad. I put my head back on my pillow and shut my eyes. "I have to take a nap now, anyway."

Within seconds, I was out.

For the next few hours, my paranoia grew. I had my sheet pulled up to my chin and my eyes fixated on the hall. Every nurse, every visitor or therapist who walked by scared me into a frenzy. Fear of someone capturing me or my family members put me on high-alert. It wasn't apparent to me that Hunter, nor Ann, weren't outwardly worried or frightened.

When the nurse took me to the bathroom, I jumped in terror at my reflection in the mirror.

"Who is that?" I whispered, even more terrified than before.

The nurse attempted to ignore the comment at first, but soon realized I was relentless in my search for knowledge about my surroundings.

"That's just your reflection," she said calmly.

"That's not me!" I answered, aghast. "She's a big, fat witch, I tell you. She's here to take me away!"

"Let's not worry about her now," the woman said softly. "Let's use the bathroom. She'll probably leave while we are in there."

Her answer made me feel better. At least she sounded like she believed me. The others here wouldn't listen to me at all. I was so afraid we would all be hurt.

My walk with the help of the nurse would be pitiful to anyone watching. I clung to her like she was a savior. I couldn't take one step without relying on her to keep me upright. Every move I made took me inches to the left. I would have walked in circles had it not been for her continuously veering me back to her side.

It took forever to get me to the toilet. When I got there, I was afraid to sit down, believing that any minute someone would sweep in while I was at my most vulnerable, and carry me away. I made the nurse stand watch as I peed.

"We've got to go now," I whispered as I tried to stand on my own. The nurse grasped my arm tightly and led me out of the tiny room, purposely putting her body between me and the mirror.

"We need to take a little rest first," she said, trying her best to guide me back to bed. My resistance was making it difficult.

"If you lie down in the bed for a little bit, I'll see what I can do about getting these 'people' out of here." Her bribery worked. Scared to death these strangers would get me, I would do anything to stay safe. Once in bed, she shut the bathroom door, taking the mirror out of my sight. She shut my room door as well, blocking out as much of the hallway as possible.

"Thank you!" I whispered gratefully as she returned to my bedside. "Did you lock the door?"

The woman hesitated. It appeared as if she was contemplating the answer to this question. Her use of lies would be limited. I wasn't one to reckon with today.

"Once your daughter and husband come back, we'll see about locking the door. We can't lock *them* out now, can we?"

If she expected this to be easy, she had another thing coming. "Those people here were not my husband and daughter!" I whispered sternly. "They have their faces but they aren't them."

She couldn't leave well enough alone. "Then who are they?" she asked. Was she trying to bait me? Why did this woman want to argue?

I hesitated. Her question stumped me. My own loss for words made me mad.

"I don't know who they are, but they're not them!" I retorted, giving her a nasty look.

A hint of a smile on her face made me crazy. Was she in on this game? Was she helping these people get to me?

I curled up in a ball and pulled the covers over my head. "You can't get me!" I taunted. "No one can! I won't let you in!"

I must have slept for hours. When I woke, it was dark outside. Ann and Hunter were seated next to my bed. I recognized them instantly.

"Why are we here?" I asked, worry in my voice.

"You're getting checked out by the doctors here," Hunter said nervously. Each time I woke up from a nap, my on-lookers appeared unsure about which Lisa they would get. For now, all around me were safe.

I tried unsuccessfully to pull my hair back from my face. I was distressed that I smelled like greasy hair and urine. I was embarrassed to be sitting here in front of my family.

"Where are Callie and Brint?" I asked.

That tiny bit of lucidity seemed to encourage the two. Ann smiled before she spoke.

"They're at home," she answered, "waiting to hear how you're doing."

"Can we call them?" I asked, hoping Ann would do anything to make me happy.

"Sure," she said, glancing toward her dad. She took out her phone and touched the screen. Within seconds she had Brint on the phone.

"Why aren't you here?" I yelled into the phone I was holding upside down. "Why didn't you come along with us? Don't you even care about your own mother?"

Hunter grabbed the phone from me before I could do any more damage. My son's feelings were the last thing on my mind. Had I been well, I would never have said such a thing. I knew that, but I felt no guilt.

But I want to talk!" I shrieked in anger. "Give me back the phone!"

"Brint had to go," Ann added quickly. "He said we can call him later."

Callie had no routine for the week, except to get up and worry. An outsider would have thought she was crazy. She was fourteen! Teenagers aren't supposed to even like their parents, let alone see them as best friends! She should be dismissing this! But what our family had was different. And the relationship she had with me would be hard to describe to anyone. We were tight! I was the one who could soothe her when she worried, pick her up when she was down, and encourage her when she needed a push. Losing me would be the worst possible thing to happen to her. A lot of other girls may not feel that way, but Callie did. She had seen my problems slowly coming on and now that they were full-fledged, denying them wasn't an option. She felt in real danger of losing me.

The phone conversation she and I had was the answer to her prayers. I told her what she wanted to hear. I was coming home! True, the conversation was a little sketchy on the details, but it was all that she needed right now. She could make it through the rest of the day.

Callie threw her clothes and the rest of her stuff in a pile and quickly showered and dressed. Each passing minute without a phone call made her more anxious. The nightmare she was living was finally going to be over! For the first time in days, she felt civil. She busied herself through the day helping her aunt bake cookies. Things were finally going to get better.

When Wanda got a phone call from Hunter later in the evening, she had to break the news to Callie I wasn't actually coming home.

"I'm sorry, Callie," Wanda said softly. "They can't come home tonight."

"But Mom said she was!" Callie protested, raising her voice. "She told me she was coming home! She promised!"

"I believe you, Callie," my sister said calmly. "But I just talked to your dad. They aren't coming home today. Your mom was a little mixed-up."

Callie had no idea how mixed-up I truly was. Telling her I was coming home was just one of the crazy things I'd said lately. Unfortunately, this untruth rocked her to the core.

"This isn't fair!" Callie shouted. "It's just not fair!" She wanted to throw something or punch someone—anything to make her feel better than she did at this very minute. Instead, she cried like a baby for the umpteenth time this week. Nothing would make her stop. It wasn't until Wanda put a blanket around her that she felt any comfort. She fell asleep on the couch, still trembling with fear . . . wondering why in the world I would have lied to her.

What little sleep Callie got each night was draped in nightmares and dark thoughts.

This particular night she woke up around 3:00 a.m. Thoughts from the day came rushing back to her. She was at her cousin's, tossed aside like a misfit in the family. If her dad thought this was the best choice for her for a few days, he was wrong. She knew she would have been better on a chair in the waiting room.

But it was too late. They were gone. She was too drained to cry, too wide awake and scared to go back to sleep. She could feel her life spinning out of control. The thoughts of my illness were eating her insides. What if I died? What if I lived, but stayed sick? What if I never came home from Ohio? The ache grew more intense with every fleeting thought. Her heart began to race. Sweat trickled down her face.

She was downstairs all alone. All the sane people were sleeping at this hour. Only loonies like her were still up and about, she thought. There had to be something she could do to ease the pain. She wasn't going to make it if she didn't. Suddenly, Katrina popped into her mind. Katrina was a friend whose mother had passed away. She had told Callie before, the only way she got through things was by "cutting." Could something that simple really help?

She pulled her shirt up over her head and tossed it on the floor. She looked at her arms and thought about her friend. She remembered Katrina's words—"it makes me hurt for something else besides my mom." That's what Callie wanted. She couldn't handle one more minute of worry and guessing. She wanted the pain about me to stop—even if it meant trading it for something else.

She looked around the living room with no clue of what she was looking for. Exactly what do people cut themselves with, she wondered. She thought about calling Katrina, but what would she say? "Hey Kat, sorry to wake you but I feel like cutting and I don't know what to use. Any suggestions?"

Instead, Callie made her way into the kitchen in the dark. She flipped on the light and opened the silverware drawer. The first thing she saw was a silver paring knife. She picked it up and pointed it at her arm. She pressed down slightly, just enough to make herself react. "You don't want to kill yourself, stupid! The point is to cut—not sever!" She threw it back in the drawer and searched for something else. She finally settled on a vegetable peeler. She put it up to her shoulder and pressed hard. It made a jagged imprint across her skin. The little teeth in the tool worked perfect. A small trace of blood made her feel victory. She squeezed her arm, watching a little line of blood appear against her tanned skin. She took a deep breath and did it again.

She made two more slices before she even thought about stopping. Each cut was more intrusive than the last. There was no pain, no guilt, just the concentration and effort it took to get those jagged little teeth to bite down into her skin. After five times, she finally stopped.

She glanced at the clock ticking away on the wall. It had been a full 30 minutes since she had thought about her mom. It worked! The effort she used to carve zigzag stripes into her arm was well worth the trade-off. She fell back asleep on the couch as a tiny drop of red spilled onto her shorts. She dreamed of knives, guns and ambulance rides. But instead of me being the center of it all, this time it was her.

Callie woke up the next morning with a million questions about me on her mind. Did the tests I was getting hurt? Was I still sleeping a lot? Did I have any more seizures? She wished she could talk to me all over again. She hadn't asked the right questions. If she could do it again, she would have more answers. She wouldn't be in this chasm of uncertainty. She couldn't bring herself to call Ann about any of them, though—partly because she didn't want to put her sister through it all again, and partly because she just didn't want to hear the answers. She just wanted to be numb.

Callie waited a few hours then gave in to her weakness. She called Ann.

"Do you know when you are coming home?" This question was the most important one. Selfish or not, she missed her family.

"I'm not sure," Ann's response was short and truthful. She didn't let on that they had been testing me continuously and weren't even close to a diagnosis.

Callie listened to the hesitancy in her sister's voice. It almost made her feel good. She didn't want sugar-coated answers. She'd had enough of that the past few days from her aunt.

"I have to go," Ann said abruptly, causing Callie to wonder what was going on.

Callie said goodbye to dead air. What was happening? She blinked back tears. For the hundredth time, she prayed this was a dream. She couldn't stand being fed tidbits like a baby bird—waiting to grow up so everyone would start treating her like an adult, someone who, in everyone else's eyes, could handle the truth. When would the next phone call be? Callie could feel the anger building inside her. Was that more tolerable than worrying? She wasn't sure.

By suppertime, she had tucked that old self away and focused on keeping calm. She probably was coming across as sad and quiet. She could see the same concern on her aunt's face. Callie didn't care. Nobody would understand exactly what she was feeling.

Near eleven that night, Callie talked to Brint for the first time since the rest of us left for Ohio. He was going through his own private hell. His days no longer revolved around his friends. Updates on my status took priority. He was worried for me, of course, but also struggling with his own jumbled feelings. For months now, he was still angry we were having him commute to the local campus for two years. All his friends were gone. There was nothing to do! Pent up indignation festered inside of him for so long . . . he couldn't just make it disappear. He tried hard to get the old feelings back these past few days. And he wrestled with how he could be mad at his mom at a time like this?

"Have you talked to Dad?" Callie asked, realizing she had only talked to him once since we'd left.

"Yeah, he calls me now and then. Ann has called me too."

"What do they say?" Callie asked, hoping she could get some information out of him.

"Just that they don't know what is wrong with her. She's still having seizures and is pretty much out of it."

Callie's heart nearly stopped. More seizures? Out of it? How did he know this?

"What else do you know?" Callie snapped back.

"Whoa!" Brint said. "That's it. There's nothing else. You knew all that, right?"

Callie wanted to tell him she was being treated like a child, like a nobody. She wanted him to take her home so she could sleep in her own bed. She didn't appreciate being babysat at her age. She knew if I was aware of the reality of things, I would agree she was being treated like a baby. She wanted this all to be over!

Brint did a good job of calming his sister down. They talked a little more about me and shared ideas on what was taking so long. Brint seemed to think it was just the doctor being thorough, and ordering more tests. Callie still believed it was more than that, like I had suddenly gotten much worse and no one wanted us to know. She didn't realize how close to the truth she came. Three new cuts got her through the night.

On July 6, they ordered another EEG.

"Not again!" I sighed seeing the cart with the electrodes coming. I had already been through one test today and now they wanted to paste those things on my head again!

"It won't be so bad," the nurse sang out cheerfully.

"Maybe for you," I said, noticing my wit was partly functional. Ann walked into the room at precisely the right time. She looked dreadful, but I didn't mention it. Maybe if she would help me get out of here instead of playing around with all those nurses, things would go more quickly around here! As soon as the negative thought appeared, it evaporated. Ann was my rock, my sunshine on a rainy day. . .

My head began to hurt. Ideas were coming and going. I couldn't think anymore.

I zoned out while the nurse attached the wires to my scalp. I imagined I was at the beauty shop and Craig was trying some new fancy hairstyle on me. I let my neck relax and allowed it to rest on the squishy pillow behind me.

I must have been making incoherent comments about my hairdresser. When I got back to 'my' version of reality, the nurse was laughing and questioning me on what color I was dying it next. I found her remark a little strange since I had never colored my hair in my life.

"Mind your own business!" I snapped. "Anyone who wears their hair like you do has no room to talk!"

"I'm sorry," Ann quickly jumped in, mildly aghast. "She doesn't mean it."

The nurse smiled sympathetically. "It's okay. We get used to patients with brain disorders saying things that are kind of wacky."

"I'm not wacky!" I announced loudly. Upon seeing my aggravation, my daughter moved closer to me. I could see the hurt in her eyes, but I didn't realize just the mention of a neurological problem disturbed her.

"She doesn't have a brain disorder!" Ann's outburst in my defense startled the nurse. The lady finished her job quickly and hustled out of the room. I wanted to let Ann know I appreciated her words, but I didn't know how. Instead of talking, I pulled every one of the wires from my head and threw them to the floor.

"I rule!" I shouted. Within seconds, I realized my high-pitched squeal brought unknown visitors. I shriveled into a ball. The bold, sassy woman was replaced with a frightened childlike being, trying to escape the situation she created on her own.

The next several hours were a blur. I gave into the unwelcome people, observing the figures shuffling in and out of the room—some handling me, some taunting me, some simply gazing into my eyes. Rather than fight them, I squeezed my eyes shut and blocked them out of my head.

Drip. Drip.

I now focused on the sound of dripping water. Questions invaded my brain once again. Am I in a cave, I wondered out loud to the empty space around me. Was I going to be tortured? Was this some type of prison where they did horrific scientific experiments on unwilling victims? My eyes went to my body, expecting to find wires and machinery hooked up to me. The only thing I noticed was a clear bag of liquid hanging from a metal pole. It had a tube that attached to my hand. Was this the dripping I heard? Were they poisoning me?

I pulled at the tube taped snugly on my right hand. "Ouch!" I cried. As soon as the word left my mouth I knew I shouldn't have said it. It would only draw them in. How could I have been so stupid?

"Good morning, Mrs. Church!"

I stared at the woman who had just waltzed into the room. Who did she think she was, acting like she owned the place?

"It's raining buckets out there today." She pulled the drapes back from the window, revealing a dark and dreary summer morning. If she expected me to comment on what she unveiled, she would be disappointed.

"Your breakfast is here." The woman's words began to grate on me. I didn't want to look at her, or give her any attention. I closed my eyes, pretending I was sleeping. But I reopened them quickly, afraid she might hurt me when I wasn't looking.

The sight of my daughter at the door caused me to catch my breath. I held my arms out to her like she was the mommy and I was a toddler. I held her tightly once I felt her presence.

"It's okay, Mom," she said, heightened anxiety in her voice. "No one is going to hurt you. They're going to make you feel better."

I looked into her eyes, wishing I could believe her.

Hunter entered the room, much to Ann's satisfaction. He must have seen the apprehension on my face. He reacted quickly to my outstretched arms, calming me almost instantly with his warm hug. I couldn't follow the words he was whispering, but I knew he was there to make everything all right.

"Stop the dripping," I murmured when I finally could focus on his face. "They are trying to poison me."

"You're fine, babe," he whispered, brushing a wisp of hair from my sweaty forehead. His touch seemed to soothe me. He brushed a light kiss on my nose. I wanted to give in, but I couldn't.

"We've got to get away from them," I breathed. "It's only a matter of time before -" My words stopped. I couldn't finish what I didn't know.

"They want to do a spinal tap on your wife," I heard the nurse tell my husband. "Has she ever had one before?"

Hunter shook his head. He looked distraught. I had heard of these tests before but my brain was too foggy to process the notion. Up until this point, the tests results hadn't told us much. My EEG showed no seizure activity at that time, but the results were still abnormal. An MRI brain scan was normal. This seemed to placate my family, but without a diagnosis, every move was just a guessing game.

I could hear Ann insisting she was staying with me throughout the procedure like she had at all the others. I knew she was there for the EEG's. She watched while the electrodes were pasted to my head again and again. She also was holding my hand until they slid my head inside the MRI cylinder. So now should be no different. But as they prepared to do the test, they wanted Ann to step out of the room. I could see my daughter becoming agitated, similar to a bird protecting its nest. After minutes of protesting, she was allowed to stay.

Two young resident doctors attempted to perform the test. What should have taken 15 minutes turned into a two-hour procedure. I was disconcerted and fearful. Ann's facial expressions influenced my own reactions. There was pain, yes, but for some reason I was more concerned with the raindrops pelting against the window.

"Tap, tap, tap," I kept saying. An onlooker would have thought I was referring to the attempted spinal tap. But it was the rain, once again, diverting my attention. I couldn't figure out what was falling from the sky.

An elderly doctor appeared in the doorway. I could see the concern in his eyes. I wanted to tell him to get these two thugs away from me. But somehow, I think he knew that already. He moved the two men aside and finished the procedure in only a few minutes. In my right mind, I would have understood residents had to practice things sometime. But today, these two were just incompetents, trying to stab me in the back. Why wasn't anyone doing anything? Was I going to be poked and prodded until there were no experiments left?

Ann was exhausted from the intensity of the situation, and I was becoming fragile. My temporary respite from paranoia was wearing off. When I returned to my bed, I flung the covers over my head and growled softly whenever I sensed someone near me.

The report the doctor handed Hunter said the Lyme disease screen was negative. We still had no definitive diagnosis. More things ruled out, but no true cause could yet be found.

I refused to eat at lunchtime, only coming out from under the covers to appease my daughter. I could hear the stress in her voice. "MRI," I kept hearing her say. "MRI."

I flopped into the wheelchair, feeling no control over my body's actions. I was being pushed around and pulled about by these so-called nurses.

The motion of the wheels and their clickity-clack were making me sick. I could taste the vomit in my throat, but I couldn't remember how to throw up. I put my head back and swallowed hard, trying to control my bodily functions. When the wheelchair stopped, I lurched forward, spewing the watery remnants of breakfast all over myself.

"I'm sorry, I'm sorry," I whispered, not exactly sure to whom I was speaking. I just didn't want to be punished for the mess I'd made. A nearby nurse toweled me off. I kept waiting for her to hit me. I squeezed my eyes tightly, expecting a blow to the jaw any second. When it didn't happen, I convinced myself this made things worse. I would be border line crazy all day anticipating a punch.

I was changed into a fresh gown and hoisted up onto a cold table. My stomach was still churning. I yearned for a drink and a piece of gum. Instead, I got a stern warning to keep my body still and silent. The tube behind me was ready to swallow me up and put me out of my misery. I longed to relax and let the situation play out. But I knew, deep down, if I wasn't alert and watching, I could be consumed by this machine and never heard from again.

As much as I wanted to cry out with worry, I didn't dare. That would be an excuse for them to kill me. I had to play it smart, act like I didn't care about anything. Then they wouldn't suspect me—of what, I wasn't sure.

I closed my eyes and held my breath waiting for the journey to begin. Where would this capsule take me? Would I ever return? My thoughts were making me sick again. I started to sweat and tremble. Where was Ann?

"Don't be scared," I heard the nurse say. "Close your eyes and think about something beautiful."

Paralyzed with frightening thoughts, I lay stoic through the procedure. When it finally ended and I saw Ann standing in the room, I clung to her, whispering my unnerving thoughts.

When I woke up later in my room, the familiar feel of the wires attached to my head made me sigh. I scanned the room slowly, praying Hunter or Ann was the presence I sensed, rather than a nurse. I was more than thankful to see my husband. Unaware that I was awake, he was staring out the window with the same sad face he had worn the last time I saw him. I wanted to yell out his name but I was afraid I would just draw the attention of others—those rude people who lived in the hall, waiting to have their chance at hurting me. I remained motionless until my husband noticed I was awake. He planted his chair at the side of my bed and talked to me like nothing was wrong. I played his game just as well, acting like watching TV from a hospital bed was our normal routine. For now, it was.

The routine at home had changed too. I listened to Ann talking to Brint on her phone. I heard the words Duke, cats, miserable, and no change. I hadn't the foggiest idea what they were talking about.

Sunday morning greeted me with sunshine, the kind that makes a person happy when she first sees it. For a brief moment, I was there. I felt the splash of light on my cheeks and my arms and legs. It reminded me of something I couldn't recall—a happier time for sure. I went with the moment and closed my eyes.

"No tests today!" my husband whispered. "It's Sunday. You get a rest."

I wasn't sure how to take his news. He seemed happy. He leaned in close and gave me a soft kiss. I stared at him blankly.

No tests. I let the words echo through my head. Of course there are no tests. It's Sunday. There is no school today. Although this made perfect sense to me, what my husband said confused me.

"I want to go home," I managed to say, keeping my voice low. My mood had changed entirely. I was near tears. "I want to go home," I said again, this time more like a fact than a request. "I want to go home."

Hunter shifted in his chair. Every moment was taking its toll on him.

"Do you remember today is Ann's birthday?" he asked.

My heart skipped a beat. How could I not know something like that! Birthdays in our house are always such a special occasion. We should be going out to dinner or having a party. Of course I remembered that! I opened my mouth to squelch his accusation. But the only words to form on my tongue were, "I want to go home."

Ann spent her twenty-second birthday filling out papers with her dad, giving each one power of attorney over me. It had to be Done. There was no way I was capable of making decisions on my own. How did it get to this point? Were they thinking I might die? Had they given up on me already?

At some point, my frightening little world became horrific enough for me to make a run for it. I pretended I was asleep, but actually I was listening to everyone talking about me. Their plans were to keep me there, forever if they had to. I wouldn't be able to leave for any reason. I wanted to scream. I wanted to cry. But my mind wouldn't let me. My only choice was to get out of my bed, get to the door, and sprint down the hall. I wouldn't stop for anyone. Who knows, by now the nurses may have convinced Ann and Hunter I was crazy and couldn't live outside of this room. It was only a matter of time.

The first chance I got, I swung my right leg off the side of the bed. With what little strength I had, I hoisted my weight on my leaning elbow and tried to flop my left leg down with my right. The momentum I created jostled my body just enough so I could slide down onto the floor.

The chaos that followed was memorable, but only to those around me. I didn't feel a thing. All I knew was that I was still trapped in this room, helpless and confused. My well-planned method of escape had been foiled. My husband and daughter were joining forces with the enemies, those *Watchers* in the hall, more and more each day. Little by little, I found they conversed with the *Watchers* and allowed them to do things to me. Falling out of bed was part of their plan to cripple me, keep me sedentary, just the way they wanted. That way, I couldn't get well. I would wither away and die and no one would know but them.

The nap that followed my fall was of little value. I awoke tense and bewildered. I recognized Ann and Hunter but had no clue about the older couple who came toting a cake and presents. Ann looked surprised and pleased at their arrival. What a beautiful woman she was turning into. I was sorry I had no other children . . . or did I?

The stiffness I received from my fall was quite evident the next morning. I was having trouble turning my head, and the entire right side of my body was covered in bruises. I felt like a train hit me. The help I needed to get in and out of bed was endless work to those around me.

My hands shook continuously now. I hadn't been able to put a glass to my lips for days. If I tried, the cup would move past my mouth and into my cheek. My legs were even worse. I couldn't even wiggle my toes on command. It was like I was in two pieces—my broken down body and my demented mind. The shell of who I had once been wasn't even a memory.

I knew nothing but what I felt at the present time. There was no 'before' at all. And the after? I dreaded the future, for it promised to be anything but normal.

An MRI showed herniated discs in my neck and three fractured ribs, no doubt due to one of my falls. However, these injuries were unrelated to the symptoms and seizures I was experiencing.

"Son, you've got to eat something," Hunter's dad entered my hospital room with a McDonald's bag. He handed it to him and gave him a pat on the shoulder.

"I wish everyone would stop telling me what I should do," Hunter put the bag down on the bed tray.

"I'm not hungry," he said. "And I can't think of anything but losing Lisa." He was near tears, He looked like a little kid wishing for something he couldn't have. The hand on his shoulder seemed to bring him back to reality.

"I know you're worried, son, but look at you! You've lost at least ten pounds. You're so tired, you can hardly function. You've got to believe you're going to get through this. Lisa is going to need you and you have to be ready to take care of her."

"Take care of her?" Hunter's words were a shout, a knee-jerk reaction to his pain. "Are you trying to say you don't think she'll get well—that I'll have to take care of an invalid?" His dad's face went white. Hunter should have known to stop, but the words kept coming.

"What the hell kind of doctors are these? How can we be here, at this huge university hospital, and no one can figure this out?" Hunter was trembling. His tantrum was warranted. Instead, he swallowed his words and headed for the waiting room, the place he and Ann now called home.

Twenty minutes went by. When Hunter came back to my room, his dad was gone. Ann was sitting at my bedside. It was obvious something had changed in that short amount of time. I had the blanket up to my chin and I was curled up in a ball. I gasped as he got closer.

"What's going on?" he asked his daughter. Hunter's words meant nothing to me.

Ann took a deep breath then filled him in on the latest.

It seemed rather than showing improvement, I was displaying a frightening new set of symptoms. A wave of paranoia, much worse than any I'd displayed before, had swept over me in a matter of minutes. I trusted no one.

"Everyone is looking at me," I whispered continuously. No amount of consoling would change my mind.

"Mom, there's no one here," Ann said.

"Sh-sh-sh! They can hear us!"

Ann just looked at me. This surge in paranoia seemed to come out of nowhere. Before, I was just scared of strangers I was seeing. Now, I was having hallucinations. I was seeing images of men and women who weren't even there.

Hunter finally attempted to address the situation.

"Listen babe, I see what you mean. Those people do look a little scary. But that's just a reflection in a mirror."

The words didn't penetrate. The wall of resistance was up for the long haul.

My chilling screams and petrified look brought Hunter around to the side of my bed. I winced, then began crying real tears when I realized it was actually him beside me. He gently rocked me back and forth until I calmed down. Within minutes I was asleep in his arms.

The scary people I saw in the mirror were now in my dreams. It was up to me to protect us all from them. I couldn't allow these strangers or monsters or whatever—to hurt us! I physically and mentally fought off the three figures for the next three hours. My husband and daughter didn't recognize the danger of them. I would have to take this fight on alone. For the rest of the evening, I spoke in a whisper and hid under the covers. My caregivers dodged punches and kicks as they dealt with my deluded mind once again.

The next day they hooked the electrodes on my head and again monitored me from 5:14 a.m. to 4:07p.m. No seizures were recorded. The results showed "an evidence of a mild diffuse encephalopathy."

I could tell by the look on Ann's face that this buzz word was plaguing her. "What exactly is encephalopathy?" she asked the doctor at her next visit to my room. "We have heard it so many times!"

Dr. London said it was a term that means brain disease, damage or malfunction. It was not about any one disease in particular.

Could I actually have brain damage? Would I ever be the same person I was before? If Hunter found this out, he probably wouldn't take me home! Who wants a loony woman living inside your house? I grew mildly agitated but withdrew once the doctor started to speak again.

"I think it's time for a PET scan,"

Hunter and Ann looked at one another. Finally! They had both been requesting one since we got here. In fact, that was the main reason they brought me here. Dr. Davidson said it was a tool that was necessary for my diagnosis. It would rule out terrible diseases so we could focus better on my illness. Why did it take five days to get one?

I could see Hunter talking to the doctor. I overheard bits and pieces. I was trying to figure things out on my own. I couldn't count on the inhabitants in this place to make me better. That was rapidly becoming clear to me.

"What will this test show us?" Hunter asked with slight apprehension.

The doctor gave a sigh and rolled his eyes. He acted as if we should already know the operations of a PET scan.

"A PET scan will show if a disease such as Multiple Sclerosis, Parkinson's or Alzheimer's is the cause. They will also tell us if Lisa might have CBGD. This is the illness I'm leaning toward."

"What is CBGD?" I wanted to know as much as my family did.

"Corticobasal ganglionic degeneration is a form of brain damage that leads to a rapid decrease of mental function and movement. There is no known cure for this condition."

As Hunter let the words sink in, I could sense a new rage growing within him, unlike anything I had previously witnessed. The doctor's unfeeling explanation forced Hunter into the nearest chair. His hands began to tremble as the words permeated within him.

I couldn't bear looking at Ann. I thought my heart would break. This awful man! I wanted to slap him! He couldn't give this to me and make my family sad! How dare he speak these words and make my husband upset! Of course this isn't what I had. He was lying! Why couldn't he make me have something else? Why did it have to be something that would kill me and my family?

'No known cure' bounced off the walls in the room. There was not enough room for it and us. I watched my husband swallow hard, then try to compose himself for one last question.

"When will we know if she has this?" Hunter asked.

The doctor looked at him with his first hint of sympathy. "After the results of the PET scan."

I could feel my family's world crumbling around me. My husband stood up, but fell back against the wall as the words sunk in. Tears began to stream down his cheeks.

The doctor left the room. Hunter ambled slowly to the window. He was staring out at the city, but not seeing it. All he could envision was the potential reality of what was to come. Ann was sitting in a nearby chair, rubbing her forehead, most likely wishing away the headache that was now part of her life. I was sitting up in bed, clothed in a drab hospital gown. My eyes were fixed straight ahead. This was all my fault. A new guilt and fear had entered my life. That last little bit of senility gave me enough wherewithal to realize I was the problem. This horrible, terrible mess was all because of me.

# Something's Wrong

A woman in blue pajamas came to take me to my Pet Place. I was getting excited. I didn't know they had pets here. Ann went along with me down the hall. She seemed so sad. I would have thought she would be happy about getting a pet! I was! It was the first real thing that made me smile since I arrived.

The lady in blue pajamas gave me to a man in the same kind of pajamas. Can't they find real men's pajamas? That would make everything so much easier!

The room the man kept me in was yellow with a big long machine sitting in the middle of it. It had a place to lie down, but it didn't have pillows or covers. It would not be comfy. I scanned the room again, looking for pets.

My continuous search diverted my attention while a woman put a needle in my arms.

"We'll just find a good vein. . .a little pinch. . ." It didn't matter. I was blocking her out. I wanted my dog.

Within a short time, I was on the uncomfortable machine. If I could get the words out, I would have asked for a pillow. My neck ached and I longed to put it down on something soft and squishy. Instead, I was on this yellow monster!

Ann stayed with me for a while. She gave me a reassuring squeeze and went out in the hall.

I don't know how long the test lasted. I just knew I was on the yellow bed for a very long time. I had a weird feeling all through my body and my head was starting to pound. I wanted to lie down on a cloud or a bed or anything other than this hard metal.

By the time I got back to my room, Hunter was there. I blinked 'hello' then waited for his kiss. He talked with Ann softly. I didn't understand their words. Then I heard him take a deep breath.

"Corticobasal ganglionic degeneration is a disease in which parts of the brain deteriorate. It is a progressive disease whereby the symptoms worsen over time. Symptoms of advanced CBGD are slow movements, postural instability, tremor, sudden brief jerky movements, speech difficulty, memory loss, dementia, sensory loss, and inability to control the movements of a limb. The duration of the disease is between five and ten years. There are no drugs or therapies that can slow the progress of the disease."

I turned to face him when he stopped reading. He didn't know I could see him. He buried his face in his hands and cried.

"She's got it!" I heard him lament. "The tremors, the memory loss, dementia, speech problems. She has it. . .This is it, this is it, this is it. . ." Those words were hardly audible. Literal sobs drowned them out.

He slammed his iPad shut.

"Liars!" he cried. "Liars! She doesn't have this! She can't have this! God wouldn't do this to her!"

Ann gathered herself quickly and ran out of the room Her dad didn't even notice. They were both in their own world of pain—each one trying to imagine this was my final diagnosis.

Hunter sunk slowly down to the floor and curled up like a baby. "I won't let this happen! I won't!" he cried. "Lisa is a good person. She is a good mom and wife and she goes to church and she trusts God to get her well."

Hunter suddenly stopped his outburst and sat up. The words that followed were chilling.

"Who am I to talk to God?" he uttered, looking toward me. "I don't pray. I don't go to church. Why would he listen to someone like me?"

The answer was in my eyes of faith looking back at him.

My husband got on his knees, folded his hands, and shut his eyes. The words came.

"If there is a God, then please help me today. Please don't allow Lisa to have this incurable disease. Please! I've never believed in miracles, so I have no right to ask you for one. But God, it just wouldn't be right. She needs your help, not me. Please give her what she needs to get through this. Don't let it be CBGD. Please don't."

I could hear him begging a being he never believed in before to perform a miracle—for me. It sounded funny, so out of character for him. For years, I'd listened to him turn down my weekly invitations to church as the kids and I got ready to leave. I saw him fluff off prayers at meals and actually tease me for teaching bible school. I cringed every time I heard him discuss his non-belief with friends who brought up religion. I had been praying for years that he would someday see things the way I did. I never expected that it would happen like this.

"Prove to me, God," he continued, "prove to me I am worthy of you. Please don't take my wife and my children's mother away. I will do anything to save her. I need you now. Please give her a second chance."

His words touched my heart. I smiled and drifted off to sleep. I dreamed of puppy dogs and kittens on puffy white clouds.

I woke up to the neurologist entering the room.

"She doesn't have CBGD."

I could hear sighs of relief and laughter but the words they used were foggy.

"You're sure?" Hunter asked. "Can you say that one more time?"

The doctor smiled, and repeated himself.

I could see my husband overcome with joy. "Thank you! Thank you!" He kept saying. He grabbed the small man and for some strange reason, kissed him on the cheek. He also gave him a bear hug that lifted him off the floor.

"Sorry," I heard Ann whisper awkwardly. "The way things have been going lately, we just expected bad news. This is so great!"

The smile that finally came to her face was pure jubilation. It was difficult for her to contain her excitement as she allowed the doctor to continue speaking.

The neurologist finished up his news and gave us a few minutes alone. Emotions of relief spilled over. We were basking in the moment. I didn't know what was happening, but I loved seeing my family happy.

For the first time in his life, my husband felt the arms of Christ wrap around him. He shared more of his knowledge of CBGD with Ann and the terrible effects it had on the body.

"I can't believe she doesn't have this," Hunter said, still in disbelief. "She was showing all the symptoms."

"It worked,' she whispered, then gave her dad a hug. "You see, we weren't wrong all those times! There have been studies that show people who are ill who are prayed for do better than those who are not." She had read all about the disease, just as he had. And, as would be expected, Ann had sent continuous prayers skyward as well.

The doctor arrived with a copy of the results for both of them.

"This PET scan is a very informative test. We've ruled out Alzheimer's and Parkinson's and ALS, Lou Gehrig's disease," he said in his doctor voice. "We have also ruled out cancer, a brain tumor, and severe brain damage."

The man paused and I could almost hear their expectancy of what he was going to say. "But we simply don't know yet what is causing her symptoms."

"For now, let's be glad with the news we got," he added." We will review things tomorrow and think about our next step." The doctor smiled again, and walked out of the room.

Ann and Hunter were still between tears and laughter. This news was overwhelming.

"Ann, this is that moment," he said giving her a hug. "This is where I felt the presence of God in me for the very first time."

Ann smiled, as if she herself was a missionary.

"I now understand what people mean when they talk about the love of God and His power. God gave me a sign, convincing me of His existence. I have the strength now to move on. I just know it. As hard as it was for me to believe, I now know God is a part of our journey through this."

I didn't understand what he was saying but, even so, his words soothed me.

"Not only that, I just said my first prayer as a Christian, thanking God for his infinite wisdom and graciousness today," Hunter said.

"Wait till Mom finds out," she said through tears and a quivering smile. Her dad gave her another hug.

"Let's read the report," he said. They pushed two chairs together. Hunter began to read.

"*Order Questions: Suspected Diagnosis: cbgd*

*Signs and History: Progressive Dementia with Uncertain Etiology*

RESULT: *There is globally decreased metabolism throughout the cerebral cortex. This could be a medication effect. Uptake through the cerebral cortex is symmetric.*

*FDG uptake in the sub-cortical gray matter, cerebellum is within normal range. No focal hypometabolism to suggest specific dementia syndrome or seizure focus."*

Ann found her words. "I don't know what all of that means, but apparently it's good news."

I didn't realize any of this at the time. Nothing had changed in my own little world.

My night was restless. More than once I awoke crying, calling out for Hunter's help. He was by my side each time I needed him, but my dogs were nowhere to be found. I needed to get home to them.

A man in a suit waited for me in his office. Was I in trouble? Was I writing things on tests again? I could feel the tension in the air.

"Hi, Mrs. Church," he uttered without looking up from his papers. I thought about saying hello but I couldn't be positive he wasn't a *Watcher*. I put my anxiety on high alert.

"I am here to ask you some questions," he continued.

I could hear Hunter and Ann talking nearby.

"Can you please write your name for me?" the man in the suit asked, handing me a pen.

"Of course," I said, scribbling down some swirls. I gave him the pen back.

"Can you stretch your arms up over your head like a ballerina?" This order sounded plain ridiculous. Was he going to make me dance? I didn't know how! I put both of my arms above my head and touched my fingers together. Memories of my ballet class when I was a child filtered through my mind. It made me happy.

"You're doing great," I heard Hunter say.

The man in the suit rattled off a few more commands. I tried my best, but I couldn't do everything he asked of me. Would I be in trouble?

"One more thing," the man said. I saw Hunter and Ann cringe at his words. "Please get up out of your chair and come over to my desk, Mrs. Church."

The room became silent. I hadn't walked on my own for weeks. My legs were quivering. My mind was tired. I didn't want to do it. I just sat.

"Mrs. Church," he repeated. "Please get up out of your chair and come over to my desk."

I took a deep breath. Seriously? Walk over to the desk. There was a battle going on in my head between 'easy' and 'impossible'. I didn't know this last question was going to determine whether I would be sent to a rehab facility or a nursing home. It appeared to my daughter and husband this show was over.

"Okay," I said softly, putting my arms on each side of the wheelchair. Piece of cake. My mind wandered for a second. What was I going to do? Walk! That's right. Walk! Get up! This man has a piece of cake for you!

I pushed myself up with my arms, willing my legs to stay stable beneath me. I was up! I did it! Forgetting the next step, I let out a sigh of relief and relaxed. I plopped down in my wheelchair.

"There!" I said. The man stared back at me with an exasperated look.

"Mrs. Church, please walk to my desk."

Yes! My cake! How could I have forgotten? Once again, I willed my arms to make my legs stand. I took a final deep breath and using only four awkward steps, I stopped at his desk. My marshmallow legs had moved.

I leaned forward into the desk to shift my weight and keep myself from falling. Ann scooted my chair up behind me, to catch me if I fell. I sat down gingerly. My legs were trembling. My heart was racing.

My family was amazed. The man in the suit put a check in the last box and signed his name. He handed Hunter the paper.

"Go to the desk and tell them to set up a possible placement."

Hunter and Ann thanked the doctor. My husband wheeled me out and motioned for Ann to sit down at the next available group of seats.

"Another lucky day!" he said. "Lisa, you did it!"

I was too exhausted to even care what he was thinking. The energy it took for me to stand twice, then take steps, overwhelmed me. I saw no reason to celebrate.

"Read the report!" Ann said, the excitement evident in her words.

Hunter stopped my chair and sat down on one of the soft chairs in the hallway. He began.

"Mental Status: alert, oriented to person, place and partially to time and follows commands. No apraxia (disorder of the brain and nervous system in which a person is unable to perform tasks or movements when asked.) Impaired recall on Mini Mental State Examination, used to assess mental status. It has eleven questions that measure five areas of cognitive function: orientation, registration, attention and calculation, recall, and language. Some paraphasic errors during exam—production of unintended syllables, words, or phrases during the effort to speak."

Hunter's gaze met Ann's. They were still reeling over the fact I had gotten up and taken a step. They were optimistic for the first time in days. The doctor's next comment, though, changed their moods.

"Recommendation: Nursing Home Placement. Possible rehab later." The gentleman's words jumped off the page.

Without hesitation, Hunter ran back into the office to the man in the suit. Ann followed quickly with me in tow.

"Nursing Home Placement?" Hunter screeched. "We can't take her to a nursing home! We don't know what's wrong with her! A nursing home wouldn't know how to treat her! You didn't tell us what's wrong with her!"

The examiner looked over his notes. Then he looked at me and shook his head.

"She has Rapidly Progressive Dementia," he said, not explaining what that meant. "We are releasing her in good condition and I wish you the best of luck with her health."

"Whoa! This can't be happening!" Hunter exclaimed. "Our insurance isn't going to allow this! My wife is not in good condition! You are a major university hospital! You are supposed to be one of the leading hospitals in the whole world! How can you just tell us she has dementia? How can you possible say she is in good condition? Look at her! She sits in that chair unaware of her surroundings. Yesterday the doctor implied she could have something that will only allow her to live a few more months! What are we supposed to do?"

"I know this is frustrating," said the man. "It is sometimes very difficult to diagnose a brain trauma or injury."

"She doesn't have an injury!" Hunter yelled at the doctor. "This is something that has been coming on over a long period of time! She didn't fall! She didn't have an accident! She just got this way! There is something very wrong with her. A nursing home will never figure it out. She needs to go to another hospital. We have to take a chance on that!"

The examiner looked at me in my wheelchair. I was oblivious to everything around me. Even he had to realize it had been quite an accomplishment for me to take a step.

"Well," the gentleman finally began, "she was able to walk a little and she does seem to have some cognitive recognition of some things. I guess I can prefer she goes to an acute rehab facility instead of a nursing home for now. They can decide from there."

Hunter and Ann were relieved, but nothing really had changed. They were all just words. I was still the same shell, planted in a chair.

Hunter finally acknowledged the doctor's choice. The man in the suit stood up, closed his door, and left.

Ann quickly tried optimism. "We're leaving, Dad. He said he was releasing her. Let's get her checked out and think about her options for rehab."

Hunter accepted Ann's suggestion. We were checking out! He went to the desk to find out about discharge procedures and getting me in a rehab. Ann began gathering my things, letting me know my 'appointment' was finally over.

My husband planned on us leaving right away. He called his dad and told him to stop over in an hour. That was the estimated time to draw up discharge papers. Unfortunately, things didn't go as smoothly as he had hoped. The insurance company had many questions.

"We can't leave tonight," Hunter said in exasperation as he entered my room. A profound coldness iced his words. "It takes too long to do the paperwork. I've already put in two hours with the insurance company. And the rehab hospital has to be a match with our insurance. Everything has to be handled beforehand. It looks like we will be here one more night."

Ann's disappointment was obvious. She had been ready for hours. She just stared at me.

"Okay," she finally said. "We'll just make do for one more night and we'll leave tomorrow. We can't let this ruin the good fortune we've had so far today."

Hunter gave her a frustrated smile. This girl never disappointed me! She had been my heroine this week—recounting my story to countless doctors and nurses for the last several days. She had given her dad much-needed breaks and had gone beyond what most daughters would do to ensure her mom was being taken care of. Hunter and I, years later, realized we never would have made it without her. She gave us both such strength and hope.

The nurses allowed my husband and daughter to, once again, spend the night in my room. Hunter kissed me good night. I wanted to say, 'Hold me! Take me in your arms and love me! Please, take us back to how we used to be!' But no words came. My eyes couldn't even express my needs. The evil thing inside me was taking more of me every day. I just stared blankly at the wall. I'd already spent any sense of clarity I'd had today.

The evening had been stressful and tiring. Ann was leaned up against the wall, her mind finally shutting down. Hunter made himself as comfortable as possible on the chair and closed his eyes. I smiled. I thought I heard him talking to God. No, maybe it was me saying the words. I couldn't be sure. I said a silent prayer on my own. Mine wasn't for me, though. It was for Hunter to find his way to Christ. I drifted off to sleep wondering what it was like to die.

The next morning brought welcome news! "They're coming home today!" Wanda exclaimed.

Callie sat up in her bed. She couldn't believe her aunt's words! She was finally going to be able to see her mom again! She didn't even ask about my condition. If I was being released, I must be better!

Callie packed her things right after breakfast and sat by the pool. She put her toes in the water just long enough to send a cool tingle up her legs. She played like a little kid alongside the pool until the call arrived.

"We're leaving here in a few minutes," Hunter said, making Callie tremble with delight. "But I need to tell you something else."

Callie's thoughts were jumbled. . . What else was there to know?

"Mom's going to a rehab hospital for a while. She needs to get some therapy. We're going to take her straight there tonight and you'll be able to see her tomorrow." The words hit Callie like a freight train. He couldn't do that to her! She had to see me for herself!

"I'll get Aunt Wanda to take me there," Callie said, suggesting it without asking her aunt.

"No, we won't be getting there until close to ten o'clock tonight. I'm sure they're just going to get her in her room. She'll be ready for bed. We'll go see her tomorrow, I promise."

Callie shook her head in angry disbelief. She wanted to yell at him, call him names, punch him in the gut! That's how he was making her feel. Deep down inside, though, she knew it wasn't her dad's fault, but she had run out of people to blame.

Callie gave the phone to her aunt and left the room. She watched them talk through the doorway and wished she could hear her dad's words. He would be telling the truth now. She watched as her aunt wiped tears from her eyes, making Callie sure, once again, she hadn't heard the whole story.

10 minutes went by before she called Brint for a ride. He had also heard the news, and was glad to pick her up. He said it gave him something to do. The two spent the next several hours cleaning the house, getting it ready for

me. They weren't sure when I'd be home, but it couldn't be too much longer . . . it just couldn't.

Ann wheeled me down the hall quickly. Wheeeeee! I was better! I was better! Faster, Ann! Faster! Why did she look so glum? We were getting away!

There's a *Watcher*! There's another one! Faster, Ann! Faster! We're almost there! I can see the door! Don't slow down now!

The splash of sunshine refreshed me. . .rejuvenated me! I wanted to get out of this chair and run. I am not dead! I don't have all those letters they said I did! My chair came to a halt. I could see Hunter and my car! There he is, Ann! Get moving!

A haze of confusion tainted the air. I heard Ann's cry from over my shoulder.

"How are we going to get her in there?"

I could see my husband running his hands through his hair. He did that when he was stressed. He did it a lot lately. But why is he doing it now? I watched him scanning the street. What was he looking for?

Hunter's face changed. He smiled and waved at two men, motioning them to come over. I instantly grew scared. Maybe I wasn't going home! Maybe he was giving me away!

Not even Ann tried to keep them from me. She pushed my wheelchair over to the curb and stepped back. Their hands were on me before I knew it.

"No! No!" I bellowed, wondering why my family would do this to me. "Don't! Don't!"

One tug and two pulls from the men settled me into the backseat of the car. One man fastened my seatbelt and backed his over-sized body out the right passenger side. The other one shook my husband's hand and smiled. Were they coming with us? They disappeared behind the car.

A man slid into the driver's seat. He looked familiar from the back. Did I know him? My eyes weren't working well. Who was this man? Where was he taking me? Panic attacked me. I froze for just a second. Ann once again came to my rescue. She slid into the seat beside me. She patted my leg and gave me a smile like I hadn't seen in days. I wanted to smile back. But making eye contact now was becoming a challenge. Somehow, I knew she recognized this. She accepted what I could give her.

I dozed on and off. My heavy head rested on Ann's shoulder. It wasn't until we pulled off the road at a rest stop that I realized it was my husband driving. He parked the car right by the door and motioned for me to stay, just as he did for our dogs at home. I watched him give our daughter a sympathetic look then dart into the nearby building.

"Out!" I could hear myself say, trying to work the handle on the door. Ann quickly placed her hand on the lock and said words I didn't quite hear.

"Out!" I said again louder. Didn't this girl hear me?

"Good condition," Ann murmured under her breath. "What a joke! We're no better off now than when we came a week ago!"

"Mom, we have to stay here and wait for Dad in the restroom." Ann's words were pleading.

"I want out!" I said again, stronger this time.

Ann tried her best to reason with me. I couldn't understand the importance of staying put. I was getting scared again.

"Bathroom!" I finally said, hoping this would be my ticket out.

"You can go ahead and pee, Mom. You have a diaper on."

Did I hear her right? That was ridiculous. I didn't believe her. I gave her a mean look and sat back in my seat.

It seemed like forever until Hunter emerged from the building. He took Ann's place, sitting down beside me, talking softly to me the entire time. My daughter disappeared into the building, just as my husband had only minutes ago. I feared I would never see her again.

Tears stung my eyes and my hands began to tremble. Why couldn't I break free? Why was I being treated this way? I just wanted out of the car! Couldn't either of them figure that out? I felt helpless. I had no control over my life. I was being treated like a child! I was a grown-up! Why wouldn't they listen? What was wrong with them?

My anger died as quickly as it had flared. Ann appeared within seconds, her left hand holding a frozen drink with a long pink straw poking out. She held it out to me, waiting for my response.

For a second, I felt like the old me. It was a summer day and I was at Sheetz Convenience Store in Hollidaysburg. My kids and I were picking out slushies for the car ride to my mom's. I had orange with a splash of cherry, Brint chose Mountain Dew, Ann sipped on cherry, and Callie had a little bit of each one squirted into her tall plastic cup. I opened my mouth and invited the sweet syrup to bathe my taste buds. Ann placed the straw in my mouth, holding the cup tightly in case I tried to take it. The fruity sensation calmed me instantly. I sat back in my seat and shut my eyes. I was like a baby getting her bottle. I had the fix I needed to proceed safely down the road. I felt the tension ease in the car as we pulled out into traffic. For the sake of my two caretakers, it was a blessing. I chose to take a nap. The rest of the car ride was easy.

While I was asleep, I dreamed about my children. I could see Callie and Brint when they were young, playing in the yard. If I knew the heartbreak I was causing them, I would have been mortified. My whole reason for living was my family! They seemed happy enough in my dream. What was wrong now?

I looked around the room. I was in a hospital room, but it wasn't where the Watchers lived. I had a headache. Every part of me ached. I was tired. I tried to take a nap but my eyes wouldn't stay closed.

"Hey girl!"

My friend Katie slowly entered the room, carrying a bouquet of flowers. I didn't know who she was at first. Her voice is what joggled my memory. I was happy to see her. But I couldn't find any words.

She talked about all kinds of mundane things while I lay there, staring straight ahead. I didn't partake in the conversation. I didn't even listen.

Someone else came in the room. It was Wanda! Yes, my little sister would get me out of here! She could stop any *Watchers* that might get in our way! And she had a girl with her! She could help us!

Wanda came to my bedside, leaning in closer to get a look at me. I put my arms out to her like a little child, wanting to be picked up. She gave me a hug instead. My pleading eyes weren't getting the message across. I would have to speak.

"Get me out," I whispered, hoping no one in the hall could hear.

"Do you need to use the restroom?" Wanda asked. "We can help you."

I shook my head no in my mind. I didn't know if it was actually moving or not. I kind of felt like my body wasn't listening to anything I had to say.

I could see the three talking together at the side of my bed. Their voices were soft. Didn't they want me to hear? Didn't they want to help me get out of here?

I shut my eyes. The pain in my head was getting worse. In my normal life, I would have taken my migraine pill. Today, I would have refused it instead. My paranoia was growing.

"Mom!" Callie's words brought me out of my stupor. She ran to my bedside, tears streaming down her cheeks. I looked back at her blankly, wondering why she was crying.

Was that my Callie? I squinted trying to get her in focus. My eyes were tunneling more than usual. When I looked at her, I couldn't see anyone else in the room.

Yes, it was my daughter! But what happened to her? She had grown! The last I saw her, she was just a little girl. How did she grow so fast?

Ann and Brint followed. I tried to smile, but my head hurt so badly. Make it stop, Ann, make it stop! You know what to do for a headache!

She looked at me with a sad smile and turned away. I could hear a person saying something next to her. I had to turn my head inches to get him aligned with my vision.

"Brint?" My first words of the day aside from the 'no' I gave to each nurse as she approached me.

Brint leaned in to give me a hug. He was tall, so tall! He must have been hiding away with Callie for years. Didn't they love me?

Ann's voice captured the attention of everyone. I focused in on her words the best I could.

"They still Don't know what is wrong with her. We know a lot of things she doesn't have, but they can't come up specifically with what's wrong."

Callie pulled the hair back from her sister's eyes. How do you know that? She noticed the deep worry lines in Ann's face. Her big sister had confronted her own personal hell this week.

"Does she still have memory trouble?" Callie asked. My daughter still hadn't gotten her composure from when she first saw me. Everyone reacted with a double-take. Callie's reaction, though, had been the worst.

Ann swallowed hard. "Mom has become worse through the week," she said. "She can't walk by herself and she doesn't know a lot of what is being said."

She was right about that! Trying to focus in on her words right now was the hardest thing I'd done in days!

Callie just stared at me. Anyone could see she was shell-shocked by what her sister had said. Ann had tried to prepare Callie as to my worsened condition, but no words could have described the unsettling way I appeared. I was not the mother she knew.

"I'm not sure if she knows who we are," Wanda said, her hand partially covering her mouth.

I could see tears in each person's eyes as I scanned the group.

"This can't be happening!" Callie cried out. "There is no way this could be true. I just talked to her the other day. She knew me! She did! And she just said Brint's name a minute ago!" She paused to calm herself. "Okay, so she can't walk very well. That's what they work on at a rehab hospital. They will fix her! They will fix everything!"

Ann's arms wrapped around her sister as the tears began. "I know," she said, crumbling under the tension around her. "Ladies Mom's age aren't supposed to get sick. And they never, ever should forget their kids!" Ann's shoulders' heaved with sobs she'd held in all week. The reunion of family brought her comfort, but also focused on the reality of everything.

"You've been through so much," Wanda said, trying to soothe my kids. "Ann, you have been the caregiver, and Callie, you've been the worrier.

Brint, you've kept the household together. Your Mom is so proud of you guys, even if she can't say it."

"I'm sorry," Ann said, wiping the tears with a tissue. "I should have called more. But when you only have bad news, it's not an easy thing to do."

Callie nodded her head and told her sister about her week. I tried to listen but it was too much. It hurt to see my kids in pain. Even though I was out-of-it, I could tell the conversation was devastating for all of them. Why was this happening? Why was I doing this to my family and friends? Was it the *Watchers* making me do this?

There I lay, dressed in a pale blue hospital gown. My hair was matted and there were still sticky patches in my hair from the last EKG. I looked tired and worn out and dazed. There was no spark, no sign of the real *me* inside. I listened to the hum of conversation in the room, not knowing the effect the words had on all of them.

Callie had to say something and touch my hand to even get me to look at her. I didn't say a thing. I didn't know if I could have, even if I wanted. I wished I could tell her I love her and everything would be okay. But I couldn't. I couldn't even return her squeeze for reassurance.

Callie stepped back, allowing her brother and sister into my little private party. They knew it wasn't me. In my right state-of-mind, I would have fussed over them, touched them, loved them. The woman I had become was practically a stranger. Callie continued to simply lean back against the wall and watch me as I lay helpless.

She could have run from the room, and probably no one would have noticed. Ann and Hunter, already used to my condition, weren't surprised at how I looked. The rest of the group appeared horrified. How did I get to this point? A month ago I had energy and love and so much more I wanted to share. It didn't make sense.

Hunter and Wanda stepped back from the group to talk. I could see how upset my sister was. She had a sense of disbelief on her face that wouldn't leave. I knew she cared. But it didn't matter. There was nothing anyone could say to change the way things were.

Within minutes, my mom showed up with my sister Glenda. Their smiles of hello faded as they stepped closer to me, shattered at the sight of my stoic face and listless body

It was Callie who noticed the problem with her grandmother first. She saw her hand go to her chest. Pain contorted her face.

"Grammy!" Callie burst out, moving past the others. She grabbed her grandmother's arm and held her. Wanda grabbed a chair and pushed it behind the stress-ridden woman.

"I'm okay, I'm okay," my mom breathed, almost in a whisper. She sank into the chair, still holding her chest. Callie looked at me. I couldn't react. I opened my eyes at the height of the commotion, but stared without caring at the crowd around me.

My mom had always been so strong. I wasn't used to seeing her sick. None of us were. Glenda called an ambulance. Callie got her some water. I continued to stare.

Ann came to my side and took my hand. She gave it a squeeze. Was my daughter disappointed in me for my nonchalant reaction? Would she condemn the fact that I just lay there, as if nothing was going on around me? And yet, hard as I tried, no feelings of compassion or worry kicked in. This action alone alerted everyone I was definitely out of my mind.

The next half hour was chaotic. Nurses rushed in, an ambulance came, and my family mutely watched what happened around them. When the room finally cleared, I could see half the group had left for the hospital. After all, she appeared to be having a heart attack. I, on the other hand, was simply fractured and damaged. She needed the attention, not me. Callie stood at my bedside alone. I knew what she was thinking—how much I would hate myself for causing this pain to my own mother. Yes, as broken as I was, somehow I still realized I was the initiative that caused this whole mess—all the pain, the worry, the unexplainable horror of it all. It all started with me.

I took my daughter's hand and pressed it against my face. I smiled at her, giving her proof I was still in there. It was the first maternal measure I had expressed so far today.

Hunter and Ann came back to the room. They told me my mother was fine and the ambulance was taking her to the hospital just to check her out. I offered no reaction. My mother was in a hospital, yet it appeared as no concern to me.

For the next several minutes, my kids tried to ignore the tension in the room. Brint caved first and decided to go to the hospital to check on his grandmother. Callie turned on the television and found a Pittsburgh Pirates baseball game. I appeared to be interested in it for about a minute, but it was only a distraction in the room. My gaze went back to the wall and stayed there. With everything there was to worry about, my mind was virtually blank. My eyes, open or shut—everything appeared the same.

Brint re-entered the room within an hour. "They think she'll be fine," he said, ignoring me and talking to the small group in the corner. They listened to his news intently. Once the conversation finished, he came to my bedside.

"You look like crap, Mom," he said, not really meaning to say the words out loud. I smiled. It was the first true thing anyone had said to me in a week.

"I know," I answered softly. Brint was happy to get a reaction from me.

I still had my wit. But the person whom my son saw before him wasn't the same person he knew. And she wasn't coming back. Whatever was wrong with me appeared here to stay.

My dinner arrived at 5:00. I awakened from a nap only minutes before. I was actually rejuvenated a little. My mind was clearer, my thoughts not so dark.

The meal was the typical hospital meal—some kind of meat, a scoop of mashed potatoes, and a spoonful of green beans. Ann had fed me over the past week. She pulled the bed tray close to my chest. She pushed one of the room's chairs to the bedside. She was ready.

"Yum, this looks good, Mom."

I watched as she put the fork into the potatoes. I opened my mouth for a second, then shut it again quickly. What if the *Watchers* had made my dinner? What if they followed us here?

Ann wasn't bothered for a second. She took the bite of potatoes and ate it politely off the fork. She did the same for every food in front of me.

"It's safe, Mom," she said. "And it's a very good meal."

At first, I tried to gobble the food off the plate like a dog. Apparently I had done this before in the last week. Ann stepped in and got a green bean on the fork for me. I took the utensil from her, but I couldn't get the bite to my mouth. The fork went first to my chin, then to my cheek. Hunter quickly took the fork out of my hand and wiped my face with a Kleenex from my bed stand. I had some difficulty feeding myself in the other place. Now it was impossible. Everyone around me could see how truly sick I was becoming. I was not capable of feeding myself, getting dressed, or even combing my hair. The monster inside me didn't even try.

Brint left the room after my first bite. Was he mad I didn't give him any? I looked longingly at the door.

"It's okay, Mom. He went to get his food. You eat yours."

Ann took the spoon from my tray and I tried the potatoes again. This time, I tasted them.

I smiled—a genuine smile. Callie gave me one back. My Callie!

After my supper was over and done with, I put my head back on my pillow. It still hurt. I wished for sleep.

I opened my eyes and tried to get back to the real world. Up until now, I hadn't said much to anyone today. My next action changed things.

"Hey, you two, where have you been?" I asked the two teenagers standing in front of me. "Why weren't you with me at that other village?" I couldn't think of the name of where we had just been. That was okay, though. I didn't want to dwell on it. I didn't feel safe even thinking about it.

"Sorry, Mom," Callie said, happy I was speaking but looking crushed at the question. "I wanted to go but Dad wouldn't let me."

I didn't mean to sound angry. I just wondered why they weren't with me then. Didn't they care enough to even keep me company on the car ride?

I stared at the two of them while they stammered their excuses.

"Save the tears!" I mumbled as Callie started to cry. "They won't get you anywhere with me!" Callie left the room. Brint stayed but remained silent.

"What's your problem?" I asked him, expecting no answer. He gave me such a look of distress, he got through to my soul. Immediately my mood went from hostile to sympathetic.

"I missed you so much!" I said, extending my arms, inviting a hug. Brint must have noticed the change in my personality. Strange as it was, I knew something was different about me—something scary to me, and now to others.

"I'm glad you didn't come along," I whispered, holding his arm tight. "The whole place was haunted! There were these people there, these *Watchers* who couldn't let me alone. They spied on me every minute. They were always making plans to hurt me." Brint took a step back and stared at me. It was obvious. He didn't know who I was anymore.

"It's true!" I barked. "These ladies, well, most of them were ladies," I said, getting sidetracked, "just kept tailing me! And they would spend their whole day thinking of ways to hurt me. But I got out before the final attack." My words were foreign, even to myself. I had no clue what I was talking about. Only the fear I experienced at that other place was real. My perception was my reality.

"Well, you don't have to worry about them here," Brint murmured, sounding very unsure of his words.

"Oh, but I do!" I said, disappointed at his comment. "They are here. I can feel it. I just haven't seen any of them yet."

Callie came back in the room, her eyes red from crying. She wouldn't look at me. She, instead, went to her brother.

"How was Grammy when you talked to her?" my daughter asked, most likely in an attempt to change the subject.

Grammy? Who did she mean? I hadn't talked to anyone since I'd been here.

"Who?" I asked, sounding thoroughly confused. "Who did I talk to?"

Callie twisted her hair around her finger nervously. "Your mom was here . . . and Aunt Wanda and Aunt Glenda and Leah." The names Wanda and Glenda were familiar. I knew no Leah.

"They were just here, Mom." Callie was nearly frantic. "Your memory is getting worse. I thought they were going to fix you at that other place!"

I didn't like her tone. Her words and accusations bewildered me.

"When you left," she continued, "you at least knew people's names and remembered some things. You're acting like you're getting worse."

I stared at my daughter. I didn't think about the pain I was causing her and the fear she was hiding. I looked her up and down, noticing only what she didn't want me to see.

"Why do you have those marks all over you?" I asked, noticing the scabs on her arms through her thin shirt. Callie struggled to hide them. I didn't ask out of concern. I asked like an innocent child questioning a hole in a blanket. I could see my daughter squirm, trying to flip her long hair down over the intentional jagged cuts. Her face reddened and her eyes showed fear, innocence, and longing. She looked at me pleadingly, like she needed me.

Rather than seek out the truth, I changed the subject. "So have you gone horse-back riding lately?" My daughter had never ridden a horse in her life.

Rather than answer me, Callie backed away from the bed and sank into a chair by the door. She looked deflated and sick at the same time.

My own mood was fragile. I wanted to shout and cry at the same time. Maybe it was seeing my children after such a long time away. Or maybe it was the fact that I had visitors and didn't even remember talking to them. And who the hell was Leah?

Ann entered the room with a can of Pepsi and a straw. She moved toward me, waiting for my reaction.

"I brought you something," she said, trying to be cheerful.

"Where is my mom and my family? I want to see them." My request was more like an order. Ann glanced back at her siblings, acting as if she was keeping something from me.

"They were here a while ago, Mom. Don't you remember seeing them?"

I willed my mind to think. Each day it was getting harder to separate fantasy from reality. My memory was getting worse. Most of my thoughts were incoherent and foggy at best. My spirit felt defeated. And as of today, I was feeling depressed. I can't fathom how I would have felt if I actually realized my mother had to be hospitalized after seeing my condition. Or if I knew my daughter was 'cutting' to relieve the pain I was causing her.

A woman in blue scrubs entered the room. She gave my kids a sympathetic look, then turned her attention toward me.

"Can you tell me what day it is?" she quizzed, waiting in front of me for an answer.

I was offended at her question. "Of course I know what day it is," I answered in an icy tone. "It's Sunday." I actually had no idea. Embarrassment struck me again.

"Can you tell me who the president is?" This next question threw me as much as the first.

"Yes, I can," I answered confidently. "But can *you*?"

The lady chuckled at my answer. "How about an easy one? When is your birthday?"

I felt stupid. "I'm not playing this game anymore," I vowed, giving in before the argument even started.

The nurse grunted something and turned to Ann. This one was a *Watcher*. I was sure of that now.

Ann followed her out of the room. Callie and Brint came closer. I was not in a good place. I didn't know my own children. It was uncomfortable. What were we to talk about?

"I'm from Texas, you know," I bleated out to anyone who wanted to hear.

"No, you're not," Callie said, unsure of how to handle this untruth. "You've lived in Pennsylvania all your life. I don't think you've ever been to Texas."

Unsure of what to do next, Callie took the can of soda and placed it up to my lips. I tried to sip on the straw inside but nothing would come out.

"It's broken," I said quite matter-of-factly. "Throw it out."

Callie looked as though she was going to dispute my comment, but instead took the can and put it on my bed tray.

"I said throw it out!" I shouted. Callie jumped. Brint didn't move, afraid whatever he did would set me off. Finally, he couldn't take the tension any longer.

"Callie and I are going to the grocery store," my son said, unsure of how to handle this awkward situation. "Do you want anything?"

My grouchy mood was becoming more apparent by the minute. "I have to eat this stuff they give me here. I would be in trouble if I tried to sneak anything. The *Watchers* could get me."

My mind went into a fog. For the next few hours, I tried to recall seeing my mom and sisters. Nothing. I would have to get used to this new life, I thought. Relinquish fitting in. Forget about what I wanted. Do what they said. I had no choice. I would go through the motions. Pretend this was all real. I wouldn't argue or speak or try to get away. The Watchers were here. It would only be a matter of time before the end anyway.

By 9:00 p.m. I was sound asleep. Brint and Ann sat on padded green chairs, staring at their phones. Callie was outside taking a walk. So this was to be my new life. My kids would sit and watch me and my husband would go to work. I would exist within these four walls.

By the time my family got home, the tensions of the day had crescendoed. They had made me as comfortable as they could. I was sleeping soundly before they left my new home. They would see me again in the morning. And so it would begin.

The next few days were draining for all of them. After a week away from home, there was a lot of catching up to do in all areas. Callie and Brint had been troopers, Hunter said. They appeared, at least outwardly, to be handling everything so well. I guess that was to please me. Even Ann told me their maturity and patience were noteworthy. The week in Ohio was hell. Theirs had to be next to it.

There also was the need to notify friends and neighbors who were continually checking in on my situation. They were anxious to hear any news, as disheartening as it was.

Then there were the never-ending day-to-day necessities—shopping had to be done, bills needed paid, the lawn required mowing. Why was I doing this to them? And why didn't I notice it? Within a few days, life presented the Church family with a new routine. My days were filled with medical tests and therapy. Nights became visiting hours for family and the few friends my husband allowed in. Ann took the day shift at the rehab, arriving there by 7:00 a.m. each day. She was the first one I saw when I opened my eyes. Ann dressed me, put makeup on my washed-out face, and accompanied me to therapies throughout the day—all at my insistence. She went home at supper-time exhausted. The physical strain and mental fatigue she coped with all day didn't stop when she went home. There was laundry to wash, basic housecleaning chores, and groceries to buy, mainly consisting of 'eat on the run' granola bars and other snacks. She tried to keep her mind on the tasks at hand during those evening hours. But simply tucking me in the back of her mind to deal with tomorrow was impossible. The continuous barrage of well-wishers and well-meaning info-seekers kept reminding her of the sorry and sad situation they all were in.

Callie had her own routine. For the next several days, she would sleep till noon, wishing away any hours she wasn't with me. She would force herself to eat something, then wait for evening to come. My therapies took priority during the day.

I listened to my daughters discussing things one evening. Every day Callie tried to come up with a reason for all this. She said she felt God was doing this to her. She didn't know what she had done in the past to cause this, but making me sick was a great way to punish her. As much as she used to love God, she now hated Him. She knew her mom didn't deserve this! The family didn't deserve this! She, herself, didn't even deserve this! How could He be doing this to all of us? And why? What had we done? Couldn't He just make me better?

"Callie, you just can't *hate* God," Ann, cried, cringing at her sister's words.

"Well, too bad," she snarled. "I do! Why can't this happen to somebody else?"

Ann thought about her answer carefully. She reminded herself Callie was only fourteen. Naturally a child would be struggling with this. She, herself, was struggling with this at twenty-two. Why not blame God? He was the one inflicting this problem on the family.

"You just can't think like that," Ann scolded. "We don't know why we are dealing with this thing Mom has, but there is a reason. We just don't know what God's plan is."

"Well, I'm getting a little sick of this 'wait-till-you-get-to-heaven' excuse, and you'll know why it happened. I don't know what his plan is, but I'm tired of working my life around it. If there was truly a God, he'd be listening to all the prayers everyone is sending out! He'd make Mom better!"

Ann didn't know what to say. She agreed with every word her sister said. And yet, she also knew, if there was any chance I was going to get better, it would be by the grace of God. How could she explain to her sister if she didn't comprehend things herself?

My poor Callie! Each evening she saw me, I was a little different. Some days, I seemed to know her—listening to what she told me and even answering some of her questions. But there were other times—times I showed no likeness at all to the old Mom. After seeing me like this on two or three occasions, Ann began to make the decisions on what nights best suited visitors. She was with me throughout the day and could pretty much predict by suppertime whether I would be in any condition for guests.

It was horrible for Callie when she couldn't come. She begged Ann, saying she *needed* to see me. But when Callie would get to the rehab and see me at my worst, she learned to listen to her big sister. Visits on those 'off-nights' stopped. It was easier to stay home and zone out on TV than fill her mind with thoughts of me hallucinating or kicking and hitting nurses who wouldn't let me out of my bed. The mom Callie knew would never do something like that.

One day trying to soothe me, Ann talked to me about Callie.

"You know what that girl is up to today? She is probably playing with her phone on your bed. She likes to sit and touch your things and even smell your pillow. It reminds her how much you love her."

Seeing her words were having a calm effect on me, Ann continued.

"You know what I see her doing the most often, Mom?" She didn't wait for a reply. She was asking me as a courtesy.

"That girl opens up your Secret deodorant and puts a little bit on her wrist. She says it's like taking you with her wherever she goes."

I gave her a faint smile. I was picturing everything she said. I just couldn't tell her.

"She's been wearing your jewelry and pinning her hair up like you always like to wear yours."

I wanted to cry. I wanted to tell Ann to go home and tell everyone to stay there. Don't ever come to see me again. It was better to leave me here alone and let me die. I didn't want them being sucked into this horrid nightmare. Their entire world had changed—neighbors started bringing food, the house phone never stopped ringing, and yet, minutes passed like hours.

Ann continued informing me of Callie's new life. "I must tell you, though, Mom, Callie has been trying to stay busy. She gets invitations from friends for sleepovers almost every night. She goes to most of them. Well, sometimes Dad makes her go, but it's for the best. It distracts Callie for a while. That poor girl thinks she's not deserving of any fun or relaxation. I tell her you would never think that. She knows deep inside I'm right.

Ann paused and just looked at me. I could see the tears in her eyes. "I hope it's okay to talk to you like this mom. I don't know if you're understanding me or not, but I'm feeling better. Sharing things with you always makes me feel better."

My daughter hadn't noticed the nurse had stepped in the room while she was speaking.

"You talk to her all you want," the man said. "She hears you. She needs to know she is loved, and wanted, and needed. You talk to her like she's your mom. Tell her about your day, your troubles, your joys, whatever. Your mom is still in there."

The nurse gave my chart the once-over and stepped up close to Ann.

"You two continue your talk," he said. "I'll stop back in later"

Ann gave him a smile. It warmed my heart instantly. I hadn't seen enough of her smiles in the last few weeks. I just wished I could give her more to smile about.

My own mother was having a rough time of it as well. Since her mild heart attack upon seeing me, she was only permitted to come to visit on 'good days'. Stress was her enemy and it was running rampant in our family right now. We had to look out for one another. Good days? There weren't many of those anymore. My best days were when I didn't try to escape or when I ate my lunch without fighting or when I spoke coherently for more than a few minutes. Those times were getting few and far between. My good days were dwindling.

"No!" I shouted as the therapist came to get me. I was to meet Robin in the therapy room. But today the doctor had asked her to come to me. I was having a rotten day. I didn't want to eat or get dressed or move. I was in the mood to cry, something different for me. I let my tears flow, hoping the young girl would let me alone. It worked in a matter of minutes. I was inconsolable for a reason no one could understand. Not even me.

The following day I was in a much better mood. Ann wheeled me down to a gym where there were several men and women in wheelchairs. Most of them were old. I tried to look closely at each one as we passed them. Were they being hurt?

Ann accompanied me, promising she wouldn't allow anyone to harm me. I believed her. She was all I had right now.

"They'll just be doing some tests on you today," a young woman said, putting her hand on my shoulder. "Okay, Lisa?"

I perked up a little at the sound of my name. Did I know this woman? She didn't look familiar. If I didn't know her, then how did she know my name? My body tensed at my next thought. Could she be a *Watcher*? Was she out to get me?

I must have looked panic-stricken. Ann quickly spoke up.

"Mom, today you are only going to do some little activities with them." Her voice was optimistic, but my heart began to race. All I could think about were the tests they did on me at the last place. They said they wouldn't hurt either, and then they stuck a needle in my back. This woman had to be a *Watcher*!

I withdrew immediately. No coercion could make me come around. I shut my eyes tight and wouldn't open them again until I was safely back in my bed. I pulled the covers over my head, showing every one this wasn't going to be easy.

Dinner was served at 5:00 p.m. By this time, I relished the fact I'd done nothing all day but sleep, occasionally poking my head out from under the covers to see if anyone was watching me. The irritating rumble of the food carts coming down the hall made me nervous. I was hungry, but I couldn't remember if food here was safe. I pretended I was still asleep, hoping they would skip my room. They didn't.

"I have some delicious supper here for you." The woman's voice was pleasant enough, but not quite as persuasive as she had hoped. I stayed under my crisp white sheet, wishing she would leave.

"Do you like meatloaf?" she asked, trying to lift my little tent. I pulled down hard on the covers, vowing I would not unveil myself until she left.

"I'll leave it here for you by your bed. Don't let it get cold."

Her voice echoed in my head. Was that a ploy to get me to eat? I lifted the flap of one corner of the sheet and verified she was gone. A tray of brown meat and crinkle-cut French fries awaited me. A+ for the presentation, I thought. For the first time in days, I was hungry. The food looked palatable. But as much as I wanted to tackle this plate, I needed to be sure it wasn't poisoned. A *Watcher* may have prepared this tray especially for my demise.

I spotted Ann in a chair in the corner of the room. She was sleeping. Poor girl. I wasn't alert enough to recognize all she was doing for me, but I could tell by the lasting expression on her face these weren't the easiest of days.

"Pssssst! Ann," I whispered loudly, hoping she would stir. I waited a few seconds. My loud whisper was not enough to arouse her from her nap.

"Ann!" I said with more force. Nothing.

I picked up the fork on my dinner tray and flung it across the room. The clanging of it hitting the window startled my daughter.

"Your supper's here," I said, pointing at the plate before me.

Ann rubbed her eyes and stood up. She looked embarrassed by her time-out for sleep, but that was unnoticeable to me.

"Here, try this," I said, pointing at the food before me.

Ann stepped toward the bed to get a closer look. "That's meatloaf," she said. "It looks pretty good. Try it!"

"No, you!" I said, leaning back in resistance.

"Mom, I'll have supper later. You eat it. I'll help you."

I put my lips together tightly and shook my head. That didn't stop Ann. She sat on the edge of my bed and lifted a crispy French fry toward my mouth.

When she saw my reaction, she took the bite herself.

"They're good," she said, dipping the spoon into the meatloaf this time. "You want some before I eat it all?"

I hated to give in, but I did. After all, she did eat some first. Her juvenile manner of coaxing me worked. On some level, I knew I was being treated like a baby. But I wouldn't allow myself to think that now. I was too hungry.

Ann fed me the entire plate of food and helped me drink a glass of iced tea through a straw. I had no means of completing this task on my own. I now relied on others just to sustain my life. The thought scared me. What if one of the *Watchers* found out about this?

I had no time to ponder this idea. Hunter came in the room with an anxious look. He leaned down and kissed me on the cheek.

"Did you eat?"

I nodded proudly.

"How's she doing?" I heard him ask Ann. They spoke in low tones for a few minutes. I turned my head to see the TV rather than eavesdrop. Did I not want to know, or was I just too out of it to follow the conversation?

Hunter looked at me with concern. "Ann said the tests didn't go very well today." He waited for a response. I didn't give him one.

"You need to do what they tell you here so you can get better." Again, I just sat still as if I didn't hear him.

"I want to go home," I said, more out of habit and longing. In reality, it was getting harder and harder each day to remember what home was like. My recollection of many things was dissolving.

"Brint and Callie will be here soon. They were busy today. You'll have to ask them about what they've been up to." Hunter's words were meant to make me feel better.

I nodded my head, trying to remember their faces.

I held as much of a conversation as I was able. I didn't feel well. The meatloaf and potatoes were churning in my stomach. My projectile vomiting took everyone by surprise.

"That's okay," Ann said in a soothing tone. "I guess I fed you too much with the medicine you are on."

Medicine I'm on? What medicine? The *Watchers* had snuck in here! I knew it! I tucked my head back under the sheet and stayed that way all evening. My thoughts were failing me.

By the next morning, I had forgotten about the *Watchers* and sat patiently, after breakfast, while a lady asked me questions.

"What are your pets' names?"

I thought about it for a minute then answered. "I don't know."

Ann just stared at me in disbelief. We had three dogs and a cat! How was it possible I had forgotten this?

"Mom," Ann interjected, "you have to remember them! You treat them like they're your kids!"

No response. The woman moved on.

"Describe your family and your house?"

That question made me sit up to talk. "I have two brothers and two sisters. My dad died. He went to the hospital and never came back." I paused like I was remembering something.

"Yeah, I live with two brothers and two sisters and my mom."

Ann looked shocked! I was talking like my husband and children were nonexistent. I spoke a little more about my life. But I shared only information from when I was a child.

Ann appeared to have had it. She went over to stand at the window. I could see her body rise up and down with sobs.

The lady left the room, obviously not caring to hear what else I didn't know. I wasn't getting better. Ann didn't even care anymore. I could see it in her dark eyes every time she looked at me. I was her burden. Her duties were continuous—watch me, calm her sister, check in with her brother, confer with her dad, talk to the doctor. . .the cycle never stopped. I watched every day. So today was probably the day she would leave. She would go get in her car and drive away and forget about me. I would remain in this hospital-hotel forever.

Instead, my daughter walked back over to my bed. She dried her eyes with her shirt sleeves and picked up her phone. She dialed my friend Katie's number.

"Aunt Katie? I need you to talk to my mom! She thinks she's a little girl again! She doesn't remember my dad or any of her kids or pets. Can you please talk to her?"

Ann handed me her phone and put it up to my ear. I listened for a voice on the other end.

"Lisa, it's Katie."

I didn't reply at first. My mind was scattered. One image in my head was this girl crying. Another image was the telephone I was holding. There was no cord. I was intrigued. Rather than talk, I kept pulling it out to look at it.

"Lisa? Lisa, can you hear me?"

The crying girl guided the phone quickly back to my ear.

"Yes, I hear you," I said at last. I heard the voice on the other end. I could picture my friend Katie in my mind. We had been best friends since kindergarten. We did everything together. My face muscles relaxed. I actually got a smile on my face. The girl beside me stopped crying. My talking must have been making her happy.

"Katie," I said, still holding the phone a little unsteady. "I called to ask you something."

"Sure, friend, what do you want to know?"

I took a deep breath and got the biggest smile on my face.

"Can you come over to play Barbie's with me?"

I talked to Katie for several minutes like we were six years old again. The conversation rattled my daughter to the core. I wasn't her mom any more. She wasn't my daughter any more. I was some lady, in the year 2012, who was getting crazier by the minute. Maybe it was time to let my mind ramble on to Barbies and toys and whatever else made me happy. Maybe it was time to give up on Lisa Church.

"Hi, I'm Dr. Hughes," the gentleman said, extending his hand to my husband. He was dressed casually in khakis and a button-down striped shirt with no tie. A stethoscope around his neck looked more like a token of his profession rather than a necessity. His eyes were kind and gentle and his manner of treatment had the promise to be respectful and caring. If I had been in my right mind, I would have loved him. I would have said he was one of those people you could talk to and feel like you'd known forever. His demeanor was informal with a "So what's been going on and how can I help" genuine attitude.

"Nice to meet you," Hunter said anxiously. "We're really praying you can help Lisa. We feel like you're our last hope."

"I will certainly give it my best shot."

Ann smiled. The smattering of hope in her eyes was easy to see.

"I've read over the chart they sent from the university," he began. "I see the test results, but I'm really more interested in what you two can tell me." His investigation into what we already knew was in simple words—nothing like the medical terms thrown around last week in the university hospital. I could tell, even through my crazy eyes, that he had my best interest at heart.

The trio went through my medical history and the wild roller coaster of a ride my family had gone through in the past few months. My decline was obvious.

"When we heard about CBGD," Hunter said, "we thought for sure that was it. Thank God we were wrong."

"I see that's been ruled out. And that is definitely something to be thankful for," Dr. Hughes responded. "But I do want you to be aware of another disease called CJD." He stopped, knowing he would get an unpleasant reaction from his listeners.

"CJD is a degenerative brain disorder that leads to dementia and death."

Ann's hands went to her mouth to stifle her gasp. The doctor continued.

"I know that this is every bit the worry that you had with the other disease. But I don't want to sugar-coat anything. There is always this possibility. This disease also has no cure, and it wouldn't be till an autopsy after death that it could be diagnosed properly. It's only fair you know the truth now."

My husband and daughter were upset, but not devastated. It seemed like nothing would devastate them now. They'd been through so much horror with me. Death wasn't always the worst thing that could happen.

Dr. Hughes turned toward me and introduced himself.

"Hi, Lisa. My name is Dr. Hughes and I'm going to find a way to make you better.

I tried to get some thoughts together to answer him, but I was having trouble with that today. My brain felt like it was strewn in pieces. All I clearly knew was the fear growing inside me. There was a cloud hanging over my soul but I wasn't sure why. I turned my head back to the TV rather than face any more questions.

Dr. Hughes took no offense. "I'd like to observe for a little while," he said.

Hunter and Ann nodded, anxious for any tidbit they could get on my prognosis. He took a few notes and questioned my husband and daughter a little longer. I cringed as they went over everything from my seizure at school, to my paranoia now. I offered no information of my own. I counted on my family to fill him in.

When the doctor left, Ann scooted to pick up her brother and sister. She told me her plan before she left. Hunter repeated it to me. Between the two of them, I kept the knowledge active in my mind long enough to greet my children by name when they arrived. Great accomplishment for me!

It was funny how a mother's love could remain intact despite dementia. During much of the day I didn't think about my children, but when I did, there was a tingly, warm feeling in my heart. This didn't guarantee I would be nice to them. I had no control over that. It all depended on my mood. Today I gave all three of them hugs when they entered and I became more alert than I had been all day.

"Hey, guys!" I said, causing all three kids to smile. "What were you up to?"

Callie spoke first.

"I've been swimming with Connie all afternoon. It started to storm so we got out. I wanted to come see you anyway."

"Callie, who else was there?"

Callie's eyes grew wide as she named the other kids who swam with her today.

"Just Maria and a friend of hers."

I didn't know anyone she had mentioned, but I could picture a swimming pool in my head. I was sure my Callie must have had a wonderful time!

Brint chimed in next.

"I wish I was swimming! I had to work this afternoon!"

"Awe! Me too!" I replied, causing the light-hearted comment to bring smiles.

"You were?" Brint laughed. "Where were you working?"

I wasn't embarrassed in the least to answer.

"Oh, just around," I said.

My comment brought a few innocent laughs.

"And what about you?" I said, looking to Ann. "What have you done today?"

The look on her face should have told me, but I insisted on words.

"Well, I was here with you all day. Remember?"

In my right mind, I would have hidden my faux paux and laughed. Instead, I became angry.

"You're lying!" I spouted off. "You're all lying!"

Distressed faces reappeared. I pulled the sheet from my bed up over my head and sulked.

Dr. Hughes must have heard my lament in the hall. He entered the room to listen in on my interaction. What was he eavesdropping for? Didn't he believe I loved my kids? Maybe he thought my kids didn't love me.

I kept my face hidden until I heard him leave. Once he was gone, I motioned for the kids to move in closer then cupped my hand around my mouth. I whispered my question, my eyes darting swiftly from the door to my children. I couldn't take a chance that anyone would hear.

"Do you think he's a *Watcher*?" I asked with the fear one usually reserved for tragic circumstances.

"A *Watcher*?" There was that word again! Brint repeated it, making sure he'd heard me right.

"Yes, a *Watcher*," I answered, waiting for their reactions.

"What is a *Watcher*?" Callie quizzed me, never afraid to speak up.

I looked at them in disbelief. None of them knew! How could this danger be going on around them without them even knowing?

I looked about the room as if I was about to reveal a secret larger than life. I could feel fear growing within me, but I had to tell them the truth.

"The *Watchers* are after me," I whispered softly, almost too softly to be heard.

No reaction.

"They're evil," I tried again. "They will hurt me if they get the chance." I could feel my husband's stare from across the room.

"What will they do? They'll hurt me!" I repeated in a desperate tone, astonished at their cool demeanor.

Ann paused briefly then asked, "But what will they do to you? How will they hurt you?"

I shuddered, not sure of what to say. "I don't know their plan, but they have one and they will get me."

Brint and Callie looked at each other, fearful of what they were hearing. Ann and Hunter knew all about the secret. They were disappointed I hadn't left the *Watchers* back in Ohio.

"I don't think you have anything to worry about here. Dr. Hughes is definitely not a *Watcher*."

My husband's words were meant to be soothing. Instead, they upset me because I thought he didn't believe me.

"How do you know for sure?" I asked adamantly.

My husband gave my question some thought, then answered me. "I know Dr. Hughes is not a *Watcher* or any other kind of evil person. He is here to help you in every way he can. I would never let anyone hurt you."

His words sounded sincere to me, but I could never be certain. For all I knew, one of the *Watchers* from that other place may have gotten to him. I would just have to try to trust him for now.

My family seemed to be pleased with the thoroughness, I was to find out, Dr. Hughes exhibited in his work. He did additional imaging, a CT scan of my abdomen, and checked me for heavy metal toxicity—an accumulation of heavy metals in toxic amounts in the soft tissues of my body. This can damage the central nervous system, cardiovascular system, gastrointestinal system, lungs, kidneys, liver, endocrine glands and bones. Once again, I came out of the tests with negative results on suspected diagnoses.

"Has Lisa had her ammonia level checked?" Dr. Hughes asked, looking back through the many pages of my chart again.

"I don't believe," Ann answered. If any doctor had checked them at any stage of this mess, she would be the one to know.

"I'd like to run that test now," he said. "High levels would indicate the kidneys or liver were not functioning well, allowing waste to remain in the body."

Within hours, my doctor revealed my levels were high, another symptom the doctors in Ohio had failed to check. This at least gave us something new to work on, indicating there may be a metabolic cause for my overall decline.

"I have a few questions for you," Dr. Hughes said slowly to my family, as if he were mulling over his choice of words. Hunter and Ann looked at him, anxious to help in any way.

"What kind of area do you live in? Do you live in town, in the country...?"

Hunter interjected before he could finish his sentence.

"We are very much outdoor people. We live on two acres in the country—lots of trees, animal life. We hike a lot too. We have a state park just a mile from our house."

Dr. Hughes seemed even more interested now. "Any deer?"

"Oh yeah," Ann answered. "They're in our yard all the time."

Dr. Hughes continued on track with his inquisition. "Have you ever heard of Lyme Disease?"

Ann and Hunter both looked at one another and nodded.

"It's funny you ask," Ann added. "My mom was researching diseases when she was still well enough to use the computer. She didn't have a lot of effort to put into it, but in the end, she told us that was what she thought she had."

"Interesting," Dr. Hughes replied. "Did she mention what made her think so?"

"I believe it was mainly her memory problems," Ann answered.

"Did she mention joint pain?" he asked.

"No, not really pain, so much," Hunter said. "She does have a friend she works with whose husband has been diagnosed with Lyme. He actually is in a wheelchair now from joint pain."

"Hmmm."

"Do you think she could have it?" Ann asked in an anxious tone.

"Well, it's a possibility. I don't know how much you know about the disease, but it's usually spread through deer ticks. An infected tick latches onto a person and can pass it on to a human."

"But I thought I saw that on the list of things she was tested for at the other place." Hunter wasn't so easy to accept the suggestion.

"I did some quick research," the gentleman answered. "Widespread testing indicated there were numerous false negatives on people being tested for Lyme. In fact, a member of my family tested negative for it last month, but was still diagnosed with it."

He paused, then continued. "Symptoms are so widespread. They can include memory issues, balance problems, even seizures. I know it seems hard to believe, but I wonder if one of these tiny pests could be the problem?"

"How do you treat it?" Hunter asked, growing more excited by the moment. From the little he'd learned from me about Lyme just weeks ago, he knew the prognosis wasn't death.

"Very simple," Dr. Hughes answered. "It's through an antibiotic."

Ann's smile said it all. Could it really be something so simple that was causing all of this chaos in their lives?

"I'd like to start her on it today and see what happens. There is still a lot not known about this affliction. I don't know if Lisa possibly has had it for awhile, and whether the antibiotic is in time to reverse the disease. But optimistically, it's a basic antibiotic. If she doesn't have Lyme, she won't be negatively affected by the drug. It's a win-win!"

The decision was made! Hopefully, I would start the regimen, let it kick in, and get better. It sounded like a true long-shot, but it was the hope the family needed for now.

They were told not to expect immediate progress. I was still my same old physically challenged self. Upon my arrival at the rehab, therapy was arranged for both morning and afternoon. But my day-to-day behavior and abilities were too erratic to keep me following a schedule. I had no motivation and even the simplest activities were complex and too demanding. Some afternoons I drifted off to sleep, right in the middle of a session. I was getting nowhere. This initial therapy, which was meant to strengthen my body and promote a return to good health, was now altered to cater simple recognition activities. The therapists worked more with my brain than my body. Simply steadying me at a baseline, without any worsening, was a challenge.

Ann had her own ways of trying to keep me in a routine. Every morning, she arrived just as I was awakening. She would sit on the bed and talk to me for a few minutes before she started the stressful process of getting me dressed for the day. She would fill me in on things at home, and always told me stories about our dogs. It was obvious, each time she mentioned them, how my attention to words improved when I heard about my pooches.

The nurse would help Ann get me from my bed to the wheelchair so I could use the bathroom. After that, my daughter pretty much took full control. She picked out clothes for me based on comfort, not looks. A pair of sweatpants and a t-shirt were most often the choices. Ann manipulated my arms and legs to dress me as one would a little baby. I didn't respond to simple commands to raise my hands or straighten my legs most days. Dressing was difficult. But my daughter didn't give up the challenge of making me feel like my old self.

"Mom, keep your head very still. I will put some make-up on you." My daughter knew I never left the house without make-up in my normal life, and I would be devastated if I knew people saw me without it now.

"First, let's brush on some blush!" she said, I let her put some on me before taking the brush myself. My coordination was so bad, the brush didn't even make it near my face. She let me wave the brush in the air until I was ready to surrender it.

"Now, for your lipstick!" This was always a challenge. My mouth now hung open most of the time. My facial muscle control was dwindling. Some days it even hurt to talk. I let Ann dab on some pink lip stick. She showed me with her own mouth how to push my lips together to blend it in. It was almost like therapy. More often than not, though, I ended up a blurr of pink splotches. It didn't matter, it still made me happy.

The worst thing Ann had to do, though, was daily put my contacts in for me. My vanity had gotten the best of me through the years. I hated the way I looked in glassed. I didn't even own a pair of glasses. I relied solely on my contacts. Without them, I wouldn't be able to recognize faces or follow the simple directions I was given at therapy. My eyes were causing me enough trouble with the tunnel vision I was experiencing. Going without corrective lenses wasn't an option.

Each morning, Ann would prepare my lenses and begin the long process.

"Here you go, Mom. Just relax and let me put the first one in your eye."

"No!" I cried out. "Why would you try to put something in my eye?" For some demented reason, I had it stuck in my head that my toes were to wear the contacts. I would protest her help every time she tried to stick them in my eyes.

"Mom, contacts go in your eyes! Look, I'll take one out of my eye and show you." Ann pulled her right eye open with one hand and took the lens out with the other.

"Now I'm going to put it back in. Watch!" Ann blinked her eye open and shut a few times and hoped that I would be easy, this day, to convince.

"Wow, it's like magic!" I responded cheerfully. "But, too bad, my contacts go on my feet." I stretched out my foot the best I could. "Here, right here!" I demanded.

Ann handled me differently each day—depending on her mood and mine.

"Mom, they made new contacts now. You put them in your eyes so you can see better. Otherwise, your shoes would be covering them up. Let me try one to show you."

Despite me making it nearly impossible, by moving too much or closing my eyes, to put them in, I allowed my daughter to win.

"There you go!" she said. "These new contacts are great, aren't they?"

"Yes!" I marveled like a child. "You know when I was young, I had to put five contacts in each eye. You guys are so lucky you don't have to do that now. I used to have to put them in, put them in, put them in, put them in, put them in. And then I had to take them out, take them out, take them out, take them out, take them out." The whole scenario would have been comical to an onlooker. It was anything but that to Hunter and Ann.

One evening I began Callie's visit with a story I concocted about a museum.

"They took me to a wonderful place today," I told her. "There were people there and men and women." I told and retold the tale to Callie, each time waving my arms and legs in the air. I made noises that resembled animals of the jungle. I was very animated and excited, describing an afternoon away from the confines of this place.

After some follow-up discussions with Ann, the pair found out I was, in reality, reflecting on the task I had attempted earlier in therapy. I was to try to move my arms like an elephant would his trunk. The therapist and I were working on sounds and movements that, in my strange brain, must have seemed animal-like. It wasn't deemed progress, but I did apparently get something from the session—a feat not obvious very often.

Another evening, I took things even further with my daughter.

"Did you hear that?" I asked. "Did you hear that?"

"I don't know what you are talking about Mom," Callie said, actually expecting to hear something.

"I can't believe you can't hear them!" I rebuked. "Chickens!"

Callie had a sad smile on her face. "Mom, there are no chickens here! I promise you!"

"I saw them!" I retorted, somewhat angry that she didn't believe me. "There is a room here right beside this one. They keep chickens in there. I hear them all the time. And I even saw one once. They are for real!"

Before Callie could get another word in, I started to bob my neck in and out, pretending I was one. An occasional clucking sound would start in my throat and reverberate through the room. The rest of the evening, my caregivers didn't know whether to laugh or ignore me. The meaning of that strange behavior, like so many of my actions, was unexplainable. The world inside my head had no limits

My ever-changing cognitive abilities were hard on everyone. Brint tried to stop in when he had the chance. He was working at a clothing store for the summer and had odd hours.

"Guess what?" I asked Brint the second he walked into my room one afternoon.

"What?" he answered, never knowing what to expect from me.

"Guess who came here and made me lunch?" I was wide-eyed, almost like a little kid waiting to spill a secret.

"Who?" Brint's passive reaction was normal now. He had learned not to take any of my antics too seriously.

"Guess!" I said again, with even more anticipation.

"I give up. Who was it?" Brint did his best to play along.

"It was the Pittsburgh Pirates!" I shouted with this look of pure joy in my eyes. "And guess what they made me to eat?"

Clearly no answer of Brint's would fit in my fantasy world.

"Um, spaghetti?" he asked, pulling up a chair.

"No!" I replied, ready to burst with the news. "Zucchini!" I laughed wildly. "They made me zucchini!"

Brint tried to laugh with me, but seeing me this way was far from funny. It took almost all his fortitude not to run away.

There were some times, though, when he spent hours with me. Was he trying to punish himself for the past contention concerning school? I now wonder.

Lunch and supper continued to bring a lot of confusion for me. Why did I eat in bed? Where was the table? Where was all the food? Why didn't they serve anyone food except for me? Brint was the lucky victim sitting today with me at dinner. He told me they were bringing his food when I got done. I offered to wait—a touch of the old Mom still in me. He fed me spoonfuls of soup until I forgot what we were talking about.

One early evening, Callie and Brint were sitting near my bed. My day had been filled with three outbursts at nurses, a thrown lunch tray, and absolute refusal to take my pills. No one could have guessed I was capable of listening in on conversations.

"Brint, what do you think is going to happen?" Callie asked.

My son was staring at me. I wasn't sure if he would answer his sister. He looked withdrawn and distressed.

"I don't know," he answered without taking his eyes off me. Rather than answer Callie's question, Brint asked her one instead.

"Do you ever feel like you're losing your mind?"

Callie just looked at him. She didn't answer.

"I mean, like sometimes when I'm home, and I'm not busy, and I start thinking about all this. . .my heart races and I can hardly breathe. I just keep thinking this is all going to end really bad."

"Really?" Callie asked. "You mean, you think Mom might die?" Her reaction to his comment was vehement. Wasn't she considering this an option?

"Seriously, Brint? How can you think that? I can't believe you even said it!" Callie's response spoke volumes.

"I don't know," Brint continued in a testy voice. "It's not like I'm hoping for it, but it's just every day is worse than the day before. At the rate Mom is going, she can't last much longer."

A tear trickled down Callie's cheek. She looked stunned. How could her brother think that? How could he dare say it out loud?

"She can't die!" Callie said loudly. "Moms don't die! She'll get better! I know it."

Brint didn't answer. He let the comments roll off. He had nothing else to say.

His sister moved her chair up closer to me, as if to confirm he had to be wrong. She stared at me for minutes. She finally spoke.

"I get scared like that, too," she said softly. "Only I don't think she'll die. I won't let myself think that. I just stay positive."

Brint seemed to let the words sink in.

"How long have you been cutting?" he asked, turning her world of secrets upside down.

She took a breath. "About as long as you've been smoking pot."

Callie's words were as stinging as his.

"I find my way to cope, you find yours," he answered, somewhat defeated.

They both sat in silence, probably wishing I would wake up and yell at them for their behaviors. I lay silent, incapable of helping my own kids at the worst time of their young lives.

'There is no wonder drug!' I wanted to say. 'You have to keep yourselves together. We can get through this! We can!'

I wasn't capable of even opening my eyes, let alone giving them advice. My kids were making their own choices without me there! Wrong choices! Please, God! Let this horrid story end! If I have to die, then take me! I am ruining everyone's lives. They don't deserve this! I could feel the last of my maternal spirit expressing what I had left in me. This was it. Somehow, in my subconscious, I decided I wanted to die. My family needed me, but they needed to move on with their lives even more. Take me, Lord. Take me.

"I think you need a visit from a friend."

Hunter's words were meant to cheer me. I was not having a good day. My stomach hurt, I'd thrown up twice, and no one would let me sleep. My arms ached from the light routine they'd put me through in therapy. I just wanted to be left alone.

My friend Rose was standing at the door. I had forgotten all about her.

"How are you doing?" she asked, most likely unsure of what to say. My appearance alone had to have clued her in. My face was devoid of makeup from sweating and my hair hadn't been touched. My clothes were wrinkled from lying in bed. My shirt sported the applesauce they made me eat for lunch. The pride I once took in my appearance was gone. I didn't even look like myself.

"I'm good," I answered, as far from the truth as you could get. She pulled a chair close to the head of my bed and leaned in to talk.

"How are you doing?" I wasn't trying to be polite. I just couldn't think of anything else to say.

"I'm well," she said. "Busy summer this year!"

Summer? I hadn't noticed now that I lived in a place like this.

"I'm going home, you know," I told my friend. Her face scrunched up in confusion at my comment.

"When?"

"Probably tomorrow. I'm doing really great. My doctor said I don't even have to do therapy anymore. When I get home tomorrow, I'll call you and we can go for a walk. I have things to tell you about the people here."

In my pre-sickness days, Rose and I walked about every day through the neighborhood. Was my mind reverting back to when I was normal? Was that good?

"How's your walking coming along?" Rose asked, knowing full well I was incapable of it.

"Great!" I told her, fluffing off the question. "But I have to tell you some things."

Rose leaned in close to hear my soft voice.

"See that tree out there? At nighttime dead cats hang from that tree."

I heard my friend gasp at my words. I could sense a chill in the air.

"Ah, I don't think so," Rose uttered, unsure of what else to say. "It's probably just a shadow or a branch hanging down."

"No! No! No!" I responded adamantly. "I know a dead cat when I see one. The one there last night was named Cordelia. She was orange and fluffy and . . . dead. She swung by her tail in the breeze. And when I got up this morning, she was gone."

I could see Rose's face turn pale. "No, Lisa, Cordelia is my cat. She lives at home with me and my family. I petted her right before I left this morning. She is fine. You must be mistaken."

I skipped right over Rose's words and began to tell her my next problem.

"And there are these *Watchers* here," I whispered, glancing up at the door to make sure there were none listening.

"*Watchers*?" Rose asked, fully getting the drift now that cognitively I wasn't functioning anywhere close to normal.

"Yes. These people are watching me all the time. They are going to hurt me. There were a bunch of them at the last place I was at. We left there to get away from them. Now there are some here. That's why I'm going home tomorrow."

I told my story with confidence and fear. Yet, Rose didn't seem to be buying it.

"Does Hunter know this?"

"Of course he does," I whispered. "They're so obvious. They might even be after him."

I didn't pick up on Rose's uncomfortable vibes. She changed the subject, hoping to find me more rational on another topic.

"Are you working on another book?" my friend asked, noticing the small notebook and pencil on my bedside tray.

"Oh, this?" I said, picking up the notebook and opening it to a random page. "No, I've been tracking my behavior. See?" I held the spiral bound book up for my friend to see. They were words in my mind, scribbles in hers.

I tried to pick up the pencil from the tray without luck. Rose saw my maneuver and handed me the pencil herself. I smiled with gratitude.

"I just need to write about some things today . . . like you being here." I held the pencil like a preschooler—in my fist. I made wild scribbles across the paper, with the dexterity of a toddler happening upon a crayon and a canvas. The thoughts I tried to portray were scrambled, just like the writing.

When I'd grown tired of scribbling, I put the notebook and pencil down on the bed. "I'll keep it there for later," I said in a serious tone, "in case I need to track any behaviors tonight."

Rose walked slowly to the window and peered out between the closed curtains.

"Don't open them!" I shrieked, scaring the daylights out of my dear friend. She closed the gap and came back to my side.

"There are some. . ." I stopped talking and motioned for her to lean in closer. My words were barely a whisper.

"What's wrong?" she asked. "Is the light bothering your eyes?"

I shook my head with frustration, wondering why no one but me could detect the *Watchers*.

"There are some people here who are out to get me."

Rose looked at me blankly, carefully considering her facial expression.

"Oh, I think it's very safe in here. Hunter wouldn't allow people around you who might hurt you."

"Trust me," I said, still soft in my tone. "Hunter can't handle them all. If they all come at once, we don't stand a chance."

As quickly as my paranoia hit, it went away—at least for the time being.

"How are your kids?" I asked, totally ignoring what we had just discussed.

"My girls have been busy with softball," she began. "Connie is really enjoying it."

"What about Theresa?" My words elicited a strange look from my friend.

"You mean Maria?"

"No, your other daughter, Theresa." I was rather perturbed she was questioning my ability to carry on a conversation. I'd known her girls since they were born. Of course I knew who I was talking about.

"Um . . . fine," she stammered, taken aback by my comment. "I guess your kids are pretty busy too."

"Not really," I answered, sounding like I was in tune with my children. "They just watch TV all day."

"Well, I've seen a lot of Callie lately. She's keeping herself pretty busy. She comes up to swim sometimes."

"You have a pool?" I asked, surprised. Her look of concern should have startled me.

"Yes, we've had it for about eight years now. It must have slipped your mind." Rose adjusted her position on the chair. Appropriate topics for conversation were dwindling.

"Jason is doing fine. He and Harold are helping Hunter with some work around your house."

"That Jason," I said with a grin on my face. "He just gets more adorable every day."

Rose laughed. "That's too funny, Lisa. I'll be sure to tell my husband what you said about him."

I nodded. I thought about asking her who Harold was, but my mind was getting lazy. I had used up the little bit of energy I'd conserved and was ready for a break. I put my head back on my pillow and yawned. Rose took my hint and stood up. "I better allow you to get some rest. It's been so good to see you."

My friend gave me another hug. With tears in her eyes, she turned and headed for the door.

By the time Hunter came in, I was asleep. My body could only fare a few hours without recharging. I took several naps through each day. After each one, my mind was more alert. I responded better to questions and I was easier to deal with, or so my husband said.

"Hi babe," Hunter smiled upon seeing my eyes open. "You took a pretty long nap. I was just about to give up on you."

I wanted to smile back at him and act as if nothing was wrong, but I'd given that trick up a long time ago. I didn't know what was wrong with me, but I did know I still wouldn't be in this place if I was well.

My husband stood up and walked toward the tiny closet in the corner of the room. It had a fresh supply of towels and the few shirts and shorts Ann kept here for me. I never paid much attention to it before.

"Don't open that!" I yelled in a panicky voice. My words surprised even me.

I startled my husband. He stopped and turned around.

"I'm just getting a washcloth for your face." He almost looked perturbed.

"No!" I yelled again, even more urgently this time. "That's where they bury the dead dogs!"

Hunter stopped in his tracks. He put his hands to his head and instinctively massaged his temples.

"Honey, there are no dead dogs in the closet. Look!"

Hunter threw the closet door open, causing me to let out a blood-curdling scream. In seconds, two nurses and an aide rushed in.

"Shut it! Shut it!" I cried. "It's too sad. I can't think about that poor thing right now. That man came in here and buried it alive last night! I tried to get him to stop, but he didn't hear me. He just kept throwing more dirt on it. Who knows how many have been tossed in there and buried?"

The women and my husband looked at one another in disbelief. I could tell they were all trying to figure out what I would say next.

"Don't you see all the blood? That's why they keep towels in there." Hunter looked skittish. I wished I knew what he was thinking. Was he scheming a plan to catch the man? Or did he know all about it and was keeping secrets like the *Watchers* do?

"My stomach hurts," I said, forgetting the dead dog story and moving on to another topic. The little crowd who had congregated at my door went back out, leaving my husband to deal with me.

Hunter gave my hand a squeeze. "We are going to see the stomach doctor in a little bit." I stopped listening as soon as I heard I was going to be checked by another doctor. I tried to pick up on the next few sentences Hunter spoke. I heard *liver* and *ammonia level*. I no longer tried to keep up with the medical terms. At the onset of my symptoms, I hung on every word when it came to diagnosing my illness. But now there was no point. I didn't understand the terminology. And frankly, even if I did, it wouldn't make one bit of difference. I was the way I was. No one was even close to changing that.

The subconscious has a funny way of dealing with things. Despite my paranoia and anxiety, the parts of my brain that worked soared into overdrive.

"I'm getting a puppy!" I sang out as soon as I saw Ann coming in one morning. "I just ordered it."

Ann returned my smile and laughed softly at my announcement.

"You ordered it?" she asked, enjoying my good mood. "From where?"

"The internet," I answered proudly. I did not have a computer in my room.

"What kind did you order?" Ann asked.

"I ordered a . . ." I paused as if to double-check my thoughts. ". . . a collie terrier."

The fact that I had two collies and a cairn terrier at home made my choice at least seem logical.

"That's exciting," Ann answered. "What do you think it will look like?"

"It will probably look like a collie terrier." It was funny how my mind created outlandish thoughts, but when I was called upon to extrapolate, my imagination was thwarted.

"Do you have a name picked out?" Ann asked me as she poured me a glass of water. She put a straw in it and gave me a few sips before I answered.

"I think I'll call him Poodle." My response made my daughter laugh out loud. There was the creative part of my brain kicking in. Maybe it wasn't all Jell-O up there.

The nurse brought in my morning pills and handed them to Ann. It was a well-known fact by now that I wouldn't take my pills from anyone other than my daughter or husband. The nurses didn't even attempt the task anymore.

"Here's your juice," the nurse said, putting a carton of orange juice in front of me. Thus began the routine.

A big pill was dropped into my hand.

"What's this?" I asked, looking at my daughter like I'd never seen a pill before. With a sigh, she started the conversation that began every time I took my pills.

"This is Depakote," Ann said, allowing me to look it over. "It's so you don't have any seizures."

"Oh," I handed the pill to Ann. She, in turn, placed it in my mouth and held the straw to my lips.

"What's next?" I asked, almost as if it were a game.

"Here's you Nortriptyline. It's for your neck spasms."

I frowned. "My neck doesn't have spasms." I could tell Ann didn't want to argue. We moved on to the next pill.

"This is Prozac," she quipped.

"What's it for?" I asked, my lingering paranoia always present at my pill times.

"This is your 'happy' pill. You take this so you can be nice to the nurses."

"I don't want to be nice to the nurses," I said quickly.

"Why? They all like you here."

I took the pill, but not until after Ann made four attempts to get it in me.

We continued until I took all 12 of the pills. The whole production took 20 minutes. It was as much a routine of the day as therapy and getting ready for bed. It was also the hardest to tackle.

"Now where's my food?" I asked. Like a dog, I would be rewarded for my accomplishment. The nurse brought in my tray right on time. They had it down to a science by now.

Ann fed me spoonfuls of scrambled eggs as I looked at the TV. She had a talk show on that seemed to hold my interest. Surprisingly, talk shows and sports were the two programs I could focus on.

"Look at that fatso!" I squealed when a large woman stepped out of the audience and onto the stage.

Ann winced at my comment. "That woman is on because she saved a baby trapped in a hot car."

"Yeah, yeah, yeah," I said, still staring at the TV. "She's just saying that so people won't notice she's fat."

Ann let my remark alone. She knew there was no use arguing with me. A nurse stopped in to pick up my tray.

"All done?" the lady in blue asked.

"Want to hear about my dog?" I asked her, probably for the 25th time this week.

The lady smiled and picked up my tray. I was stuck on the dog topic. If I talked about dogs in the morning, the topic stayed with me all day, sometimes for many days,

One afternoon, Ann and Callie were sitting with me after a tough therapy session. When I'd returned to my room, I lay my head back and closed my eyes.

"Help me, I'm drowning!" I said with my eyes still closed. "I'm a little pink poodle, save me!" I made flailing motions with my arms as if I was the one in trouble.

My two daughters just sat back and looked at me. I didn't know what they were thinking, but it had to be thoughts of sadness and hopelessness. Where had their mom gone, and would she ever come back?

Most of the time, my days ran together. Today was a little different.

"Remember the problems you've always had with your neck?" Ann asked me one afternoon after lunch. "On the MRI you had in Ohio, it showed you have some herniated discs. You need to go see a doctor about it today."

I sat despondent in my bed. She was mainly telling me about the tests out of respect. If I had been in my right mind, I would have wanted to know all the information I could get. She knew that. She did her best to explain the unexplainable.

Some days I chattered nonstop, but I had days like today just as often. I was zoned out. I wasn't paying attention to anything around me. Ann was trying to prep me for my side trip to the doctor today. It wouldn't have mattered if she said we were going to Disneyland. I wasn't going to react.

The doctor confirmed there was disc damage but nothing needed attention right away. After all, when you are in full-blown dementia, a pain in the neck is the least of your problems. Due to the therapy, though, it was important to make sure I wasn't damaging anything else in the few minutes of exercise I did get.

"I'm going away for a few days," Dr. Hughes mentioned when he stopped to check on me that afternoon. "I want to make sure Lisa is stable before I go." It was obvious he was continuing to give my case a lot of time and thought.

"First," he began, "I would like to take Lisa off two drugs that she's been on for a few years now. They are for her blood pressure and muscle spasms. I really want to cleanse her system. Being without them will not harm her."

Ann nodded her head in agreement.

"I also want to decrease her Depakote dosage slightly and put her back on Topomax. With these changes, and the addition of the antibiotic for

Lyme disease, I feel pretty confident we should see a positive change in Lisa by the time I return." My family was beside themselves with anticipation and fear. . .afraid to hope, afraid not to.

This was finally Ann's chance to take a breath and think positively for a while. She hadn't allowed herself to feel anything but worry over the past two months. I was getting sleepy, so my naptime was her work time.

The list she had in front of her was a mile long! She rarely left me during the day. She'd neglected numerous errands and activities that required her attention. She was hoping to sneak out during one of my naps. Her phone buzzed just as I was getting sleepy.

"Yes, yes, that's not a problem. That will be fine! Thanks so much!"

Ann hung up the phone just as her dad walked in.

"Wow, I haven't seen a smile like that in awhile," he said. "What's up?"

"I got an interview at the high school!" she blurted out. "I've got an interview!" This was the call she'd been waiting for! How I wished I was alert enough to share in her excitement!

Hunter moved toward her and gave her a big hug. Tears were in his eyes. This feeling of jubilation should have swept her away. But then she saw me.

The look on her face was one of devastation and guilt.

"What am I thinking?" she asked, dabbing at the tears now running down her cheeks. "I can't take on a job with Mom like this!" Her words were not mean or unkind. They were matter-of-fact. What seemed to be the most important thing in her world just a few weeks ago now was a hassle, something that just needed to be crossed off her list.

I wanted her to keep her mind on the good news. She should be wondering what she would wear and what will they ask! She should be asking me for advice, not worrying about my life in the coming months. I could tell by the look on her face she had already decided a teaching job was not in her plans right now. She would be taking care of me this fall, not teaching in her own classroom. She would be a servant catering to my every need.

"You're going to that interview," Hunter said, brushing a tear from her cheek. "Do you know how disappointed Mom would be if you didn't take advantage of this?"

"But Dad. . ." she continued.

"There are no buts," he said. "You have worked toward this your entire life. To be a teacher is a dream of yours just like it was for your mom and me. If she were to find out you weren't pursuing it. . .especially because of her, she would be crushed."

"I know," my daughter said softly.

"And Dr. Hughes said she should be improving soon." Hunter tried to sound hopeful, but he knew I was not improving. I was getting worse. Chances of me being in a nursing home in the fall were not only plausible, but probable.

"I'll go to the interview," Ann said, "just for the experience. But if I'm offered the job and Mom isn't better then—"

"We'll talk about it then," Hunter interrupted, as if speaking of my demise would make it certain.

There were a million questions I wanted to ask! Would she be teaching in a local school, coming home to help me with supper, happy as could be? Or would there be a hospital bed in our den—with Ann having a full-time job taking care of me and the household? I squelched the thought by closing my eyes tightly. I didn't even want to imagine that! And yet, I couldn't help but think about it in my few private, lucid moments.

Ann spent the next few hours brainstorming. The interview was in two days. I could hear Hunter and her talking about my schedule, and who would sit with me when. Oh, why did it have to be this way? Once again, I was ruining something important to my family. I wished with all my might I could rid her mind of the turmoil going on around her. But there was no use. I couldn't do anything to help. My illness brutally touched everyone I loved.

For the first time, Hunter was truly falling apart. Thinking about Ann's job interview really got him thinking. Up until now, everything was in a holding pattern. Things were always 'when Lisa gets better'. Now, he was being forced to think about me *not* getting better. What would he do if faced with that scenario? Keep me at home and hire someone to stay with me? Retire early and take care of me himself? Put me in a nursing home and pledge it was only for a little while? Every time he tried to face the issues, he retreated to a place deep within, and tried to convince himself this wasn't going to happen. But time was running out. It would be better to have things planned out, rather than have to make a snap decision.

Either way, he needed to stop worrying for a few hours. If he didn't, he wasn't sure how he would face another day.

As always, Hunter waited until I was asleep before he left me for the night. He picked up his keys and headed for the parking lot.

He just couldn't go home yet. He watched the second-shift nurses scatter in the parking lot. How he envied anyone tonight who could just go home to a normal life. He'd all but forgotten how that felt.

Two of the nurses he'd seen before gave him a wave. "You're welcome to join us if you need a beer," one said. He had recognized them from the rehab. They weren't caregivers of mine, but they were in the next unit.

How thoughtful, he mused. His first reaction was to just wave them off and yell good-night. But then he recalled how harrowing the last few days had been. What could one beer hurt? He would have a drink, talk with the girls, and be home in an hour. Maybe the pain would lessen a little, or his outlook on life wouldn't be so dismal. It was worth a try.

He followed their car to a local bar tucked in on a back street. He'd forgotten this place even existed. He'd been to it maybe once or twice before he was married. It was a neighborhood bar that catered to the locals. Good, he thought. He wouldn't see anyone he knew. He could blend in with the scenery for a while then head home.

The two girls from the rehab jumped out of the car eagerly. They waited for Hunter to catch up.

"Ever been here before?" one asked, rummaging through her purse for her lipstick. "I'm Gretchen, by the way, and this is Eve."

"Hunter," my husband said, "Nice to meet you. I've talked to so many inside that hospital I'm not sure who I know and don't know."

"We've seen you around," Eve said, unclipping the name tag from her scrubs. "Sorry to hear about your wife."

Hunter put his head down. For the first time in months, he had actually forgotten the horrible situation he was in. It was short-lived.

"Thanks," he said, holding the door open for the two of them. He made a promise to himself he wasn't going to even bring me up. This was his diversion, a distraction away from the misery and sadness he felt all the time. A reprieve would be nice—even a short one.

They sat down at the end of the bar. He put down a $20 and told them to order what they wanted. He got himself a Coors LIGHT. For just a moment, he allowed himself to relax. He shut his eyes and took a deep breath. Maybe this whole lousy world would be gone when he opened them. He heard the bartender put a bottle on the bar. He sighed, knowing everything was still too real to cope with.

Gretchen saw a group of friends at a nearby table. She nudged Eve, letting her know where she was off to. Eve didn't seem to mind. She stirred her rum and coke and adjusted her stool within talking distance of Hunter.

"You okay?" she asked.

Hunter nodded his head. "Long day."

"It's a rough case," she whispered, knowing all too well the dire scenario of how things turned out for a lot of the patients she cared for. "I wish I could say something to make you feel better . . . ."

Her words piqued his interest.

"Thanks." The woman's words were meant to help, but he found no consolation in them. In fact, Hunter was almost irritated. But then he caught himself... his anger toward the world right now was not her problem. How he felt—the bitterness, the exhaustion, the fury he had welled up inside of himself—none of it was her fault. He had no right to share any of his raw emotions with her.

The woman must have recognized his turmoil. She put her hand on his shoulder and gave it a comforting squeeze. Her gaze stayed on him as he felt a tear run down his cheek. He put his head down, hoping she wouldn't notice.

"I think you could use someone to talk to," she said. Hunter couldn't bring himself to look at her. Instead, he put his hand up, trying to brush off her suggestion.

"Come on, follow me," she said, taking his beer with her. As much as he didn't want to, he followed her. She led them onto the patio.

"It's a little easier to talk out here," she said.

They sat down in the corner, away from the others who all appeared to be having a good time. How he envied them. How he wished it was last summer at this time, and this whole nightmare wouldn't have started yet. Maybe he could even have prevented it from happening.

"I'm sorry," he found himself saying. "You've caught me at a bad time. I'm usually not one to crumble, but things just aren't going well. I haven't let myself get to this point yet. I've had to be strong for the kids, but to be honest, I don't think I can do it anymore."

"You can and you will," the nurse said in a positive tone. She was pretty. She was calming. She was exactly what he needed right now.

"I can't even begin to tell you how this whole thing started," Hunter said in almost a whisper. "It was like, one day things were fine, and the next, my wife is out of her mind. It's just hard to grasp. I can't get past seeing her strapped down to the bed, shouting nonsense things at her kids and you nurses. It's just not Lisa."

"I know," Eve uttered in her soothing voice. "You have to keep faith she'll come back to you soon. Things will get back to normal."

The nurse was lying and Hunter knew it. There was no way I could snap out of this and become my regular self again. It was too late. There was already some brain damage, the doctor had said so. Even if I came out of this stupor right now, I would never be the same. No, the Lisa who Hunter knew and loved so much was already gone.

Hunter swigged down his beer and ordered another one. Eve had another rum and coke and both of them began to relax. Hunter hadn't felt relief like this in ages. Having someone to talk to was great. Doing it over a few beers was better. He took off his glasses and rubbed his eyes. The combination of smoke and the heat of the night made his eyes tear.

"So, I guess you've seen a lot of different cases in your time here?" Hunter asked his new friend, trying to be polite and get away from his own story for a while.

She smiled. It was a sweet smile, not a fake one. He could instantly sense the warmth.

"Oh yes, I have seen a lot in my ten years at the rehab. In fact, I've seen miracles more than once."

Her last words echoed in Hunter's mind. Miracles? That's what this case would take—a miracle.

"So . . . they happen?" Hunter asked, intrigued.

"They certainly do, Hunter. I've seen paralyzed people walk out of the hospital. I've seen victims of car crashes go from a hopeless mess back to the families they love. There is always reason to hold out for a miracle. And as far as doctors go, you could not ask for anyone better than Dr. Hughes. He has a reputation that is unmatched in this area. He knows his stuff. And he's constantly reading up on things and going to conferences. Yes, there are times when circumstances prevent a full recovery. But Dr. Hughes has a way of taking a person to the highest level he or she can reach. And I'm sure, in Lisa's case, she has a great shot at getting out of the hospital and home to the family she loves."

Hunter chugged a little more of his beer, liking what she was saying. From everything he'd read and heard, Dr. Hughes did appear to be the best of the best. Hunter needed to be optimistic. He couldn't let broken days like today crush him.

He asked for another beer, almost daring himself to laugh in the face of fate. He took a swallow and shut his eyes. He could feel his mind go a little numb. He wanted to feel guilty about his lack of discretion, but he wouldn't let that thought intrude. He needed some "me" time. He was going to break if he didn't get it.

Massaging his temples, Hunter could almost make his problem disappear. He stared at the TV in the corner of the patio, then looked back over to Eve. The sights and sounds around him were taking him almost into a twilight zone. Here he was, sitting in a bar with an attractive woman, so far removed from hospital beds and therapy exercises and hallucinatory conversation. He liked it here. He liked that feeling. He liked the idea of making it never end.

They sat there for hours, talking about sports, books, and even the weather. The only subject taboo was the rehab. By two a.m. he was drunk. So was Eve. When she gave him that sexy smile, he knew there was no turning back. He had had too many beers and allowed the loneliness in his heart to take over. He leaned in across the table and took her face in his hands. The kiss that followed was captivating.

He hadn't kissed another woman in over 30 years. The taste of her lipstick, the fresh smell of her hair, it was all so new and exciting for him. He leaned back and looked into her eyes. She obviously felt the same way. Without thinking, Hunter threw cash on the table and grabbed her hand. He headed for the back door, with her close behind. He wasn't sure where they would end up.

When they finally got out of the building, Hunter scanned the area to get his bearings. He expected to come out into the darkness. Instead, he was at the edge of the outdoor tables. A few couples were seated, another group of guys was congregated in the corner, drinking beers and telling stories. There was no privacy.

Hunter turned around to make sure Eve was still coming. She gave him a smile, more of a giggle, actually, and pointed to the parking lot. Hunter could feel the keys jingling in his pocket. He pulled them out and unlocked the doors. But instead of getting in, Eve tugged at his arm.

"I live right over here," she whispered. Hunter gave a quick sigh of relief then allowed the excitement to take over again. He followed her into her house and down the hall. He was ready. He needed this!

Eve made a left at the end of the hall into a large bedroom. He followed her in. The first thing he saw was an antique oak sleigh bed. Hunter stopped. He just looked at it. His head was spinning, but he took in the view of the lovely country furnishings.

"It's a bed, silly," Eve laughed at his hesitation. "Get your clothes off and join me in it."

"My wife would love this bed," he said, inebriated, looking at it in awe. "This whole room—she would absolutely love it." He spoke as if Eve wasn't even there.

The woman looked at him. She allowed the rum and coke to talk.

"Seriously?"

Hunter didn't take the sarcastic remark as she meant it.

"Yes," Hunter answered, totally taken aback. "She has been looking for one like this for years."

He sat down on the edge of it, and touched the smooth wood. He looked slowly about the room. His real-life situation and the day he had flashed in his mind. Thank God he realized the mistake he had been about to make. He shook his head. He couldn't believe he had allowed himself to get so drunk. He really couldn't believe he had followed Eve home. This was not like him at all. In thirty-two years of marriage, he had never once been tempted to cheat. What was he doing? How could things have even gone this far?

"This isn't gonna happen, is it?" Eve asked, sitting down on the other side of the bed.

"No. I'm sorry Eve. I don't know what to say. I just let things get out of hand. You are so pretty and nice and I really liked talking to you. But I love Lisa. . .so much. I can't believe I almost actually messed things up. She is sick. She needs me. I need her. . ."

Eve let him ramble on until tears filled his eyes. That was what he needed—someone to listen to him—not sex. He was so, so glad he had stopped.

"You can stay here until you sober up," Eve offered. "I'm going to shower and get to bed. I have to work again tomorrow."

"Thanks," Hunter answered. Suddenly he remembered he hadn't checked his phone in hours. What if the hospital called? What if the kids needed him? Just another part to this whole horrid predicament he'd created for himself! He reached into his pocket and felt for his phone. It wasn't there. He checked his other pockets and stood up to search where he was sitting. Nothing.

"Have you seen my phone?" he asked. He was starting to get worried. It wasn't like him these days, to lose track of where he put it.

"I think you threw it in your car when you thought we were getting in."

Was he really that thoughtless tonight, he said to himself.

He left the house and looked around for where he was parked. His senses were all coming back slowly. This was definitely sobering him up. He spotted his car and raced to it, praying his phone would be safely on his seat. It was.

Hunter heaved a sigh of relief and picked it up. 10 missed calls—8 from the hospital and 2 from Brint! Dammit! Hunter called himself a few choice words. What did he expect? He was asking for problems when he thought he could just walk away from everything!

Any other night, he would have been home by now, getting the few hours of sleep he needed to keep going. He also would have answered his phone!

"Mr. Church?"

"Yes," he stuttered, feeling shame and worry mixed together in a ball in the pit of his stomach.

"I'm sorry to interrupt you." Hunter hated the way she said it. Interrupt. What a word.

The voice on the other end of the line let him know the problem.

"Your wife is unresponsive, Mr. Church. We've been trying to call you. They just loaded her up for the hospital."

They couldn't wake her up? Why did she need to get up? It was the middle of the night! He wanted to ask questions. Instead, he said he'd meet them at the hospital.

He started out for the hospital, condemning his actions the entire way. His wife could be dying and he'd almost been in the arms of another woman! He was physically sick. He swallowed the vomit he felt in his throat. He thought of Eve, for an instant. He definitely couldn't blame things on her! He was the one at fault here.

He thought of calling Brint but decided against it. He was probably asleep. He had Ann's number punched in, but hung up instead of letting the call go through. She most definitely would be in bed by now. There was no need to wake her up until he knew something. He scanned the neighborhood, glad that Eve's neighbors were in bed. He was embarrassed and angry—an unpleasant combination.

He made a left at the stop sign and took a deep breath. You can get past this, he kept telling himself. He shook his head like the fool that he was and kept going.

Unaware of my situation, Ann was finally enjoying an evening out and away from the worries of her world. At first, she couldn't relax. She felt like she was doing something wrong, turning her back on me. But once she told herself it was okay to set aside the worry for one night, she allowed herself to enjoy the company of a friend. Trevor and she went from the bar to his house, talking about anything and everything . . . except me. It was nearly 4:00 a.m. when Trevor took her home. Her heart sank when she realized her dad's car was not in the driveway. There was only one place he could be. She thanked Trevor and got out of the car. Callie met her at the door.

"Where have you been?" Callie asked, terror in her eyes.

Ann ignored the chastising and moved on to what really mattered.

"Is Dad at the hospital? What happened?" Her mouth was moving but she could barely utter what was coming out. She never should have gone out! What was wrong?

"They called a couple of hours ago, but wouldn't say what was going on. Brint tried to call Dad, but he wouldn't answer his phone. We've been trying and trying to call you. Why didn't you answer?"

Ann's vow to not look at her phone that night was coming back to bite her.

Callie was crying by this time. She had needed her sister and she wasn't there for her. Neither was her dad.

"It's okay," Ann said, giving her sister a hug. "I'll find out what's going on."

In my own fantasyland that same night, my thoughts were more jumbled and frantic than anyone's. I had gone to bed as usual that evening. Hunter gave me a kiss goodbye on his way out the door. He thought I was asleep, but I had no plans for sleeping tonight.

The first *Watcher* came in just a few minutes after my husband left. She pretended to be nice to me, but I kept my eyes closed so she would leave. She didn't. She walked around the room. I could hear her but I didn't know what she was doing. My mind took over and let me know just what was going on.

The instant I heard her open that closet door, I knew I was in for a night of terror. She was searching for the dead dogs.

My next thought startled me like none other! Were *my* dogs in there? It was almost too horrific to think about. But I wonder if that's how I know about the dead dogs? Did that closet have in all the dogs I ever had in my whole life? There would be a lot—Tammy, Spot, Gerta, Jingles, Bridget, Rusty, Heidi, Maggie, Ginger, Daisy. . .oh no! What if they killed my dogs that live at my house? Please no, not my Duke!! He is bad sometimes but I love him. . .so much.

But if *my* old dogs are in there, then what would be in the closets where my brothers and sisters slept? They were their dogs too. Did the *Watchers* cut the dogs up in pieces and give some to everybody? What parts did I get?

"Lisa, open your eyes." The lady said it so sweetly. Did she think I would fall for that?

I felt her come in closer.

"Come on, Lisa. I need for you to get awake. The doctor wants me to give you this pill."

Pill! Good try, lady. I know every pill I get in this place. And I don't need one from you!

"Come on. Get awake!" She was now tapping me on the shoulder. Tap, tap, tap. She must be the one from the other place. I can remember. Tap, tap, tap. The *Watchers* at that other place hurt me when they said that. Tap, tap, tap. I couldn't let that happen to me again. I wasn't going to roll over and let them stick that big needle in me again!

I heard the *Watcher* in a different spot in the room. I heard her. Splash. Splash. Splash. What was she doing now? I heard her one more time. Splash. Splash. Splash. Then I heard her walk over to me again. I kept my eyes closed, praying she wouldn't hurt me.

It was then I felt the blood. She was wiping blood on my face. She was using a soft cloth to wipe blood from the dead dogs on my face.

"This will get you up," I heard her sing softly.

She wiped the blood on my forehead and my cheeks and my nose. It was cold. It was wet. She kept on saying 'This will get you up. Yes, this will get you up.' She even wiped it on my arms.

I stayed as still as I could. I pretended I was fast, fast asleep. After just a few seconds more, my bloody bath stopped. The *Watcher* simply took her bloody cloth and left.

I was still too afraid to open my eyes. What if she wants me to think that she left, but she didn't? No, I would keep my eyes shut forever if I had to. I almost fell asleep while I was waiting. But a noise at the door made my mind stay awake. Still, I was a good girl—I kept my eyes closed.

I felt them as they lifted me off my bed and onto another. This one had wheels! Where were they taking me? I wanted to open my eyes, open my eyes, open my eyes. I couldn't.

I felt myself being wheeled down a hall quickly. It was only a matter of minutes and I was in the hearse. It was taking me away.

"Lisa?"

I heard my name!

"You're in an ambulance, Lisa." The man's tone scared me a little. He sounded frustrated and demanding at the same time. I felt the need to keep the conversation going.

"What's wrong with me?" I asked, expecting him to tell me some outlandish lie.

"You were unresponsive," he answered, looking over at a machine that was making noises.

Unresponsive! What did that mean?

"I was not!" I barked. I prayed the *Watcher* wouldn't get angry because I argued with him.

"You were unresponsive, Lisa, but you seem to be responding now."

"I'm sorry, I'm sorry!" I whispered. The man paid no attention to my words. He made a phone call, telling someone, probably another *Watcher*, that he had me.

"Should I still bring her in?" I heard him say softly, most likely so I wouldn't hear.

Bring me in? Where was he taking me?

"I want to go back!" I cried, unable to control my urge to speak.

He hung up the phone, or whatever the thing was he was talking into, and looked my way.

"We're still taking you to the hospital, Lisa, to get you checked out." His words hit me like a slap across my face.

I tried to kick the man but my legs were strapped down. I curled my hands into fists with plans to hit him. He saw my antagonized state and grabbed them before I could make contact.

"They said you may get like this!" the perturbed man uttered. "I should have done this before we left." He took the dangling strap and tightened it across my chest. I cried out in rage, anticipating our arrival in Ohio any minute. Having no other means to get away, I spit on the man, trying to get his attention away from me.

"You're mean!" I yelled, knowing my attempt at spitting was laughable. I couldn't spit anymore than I could punch, hit, or kick him. "You'll be sorry!" I groaned, arching my back in one last feeble attempt to get up. "I'll get you in trouble for this!"

My outburst had no effect on him. I took a deep breath and tilted my neck so I could see myself positioned on the stretcher. They were no straps that I could see holding me in, no look of distress on the man beside me. It was all in my mind, I tried to tell myself. But I couldn't be sure.

I felt the ambulance lurch to a halt in front of a huge white building. "We're here, Lisa," I heard the *Watcher* say. "You're going to be fine. They'll take good care of you."

The attendant quickly wheeled me into the hospital. I was pleading with my eyes to every person we passed. No one was paying attention.

The medics wheeled me in through the ambulance entrance. I was still on the gurney, but was sitting up alert and aware of my surroundings.

It seemed like forever, but Hunter arrived just minutes after they brought me in.

"She perked up shortly after we left the rehab," the young medic told Hunter.

"Why am I in the hospital?" I asked, thinking immediately of the *Watchers* who lived in these places.

"You were unresponsive," Hunter said, not knowing if I would know what that term meant.

"What?" I asked, a puzzled and somewhat irritated look on my face.

"The nurses couldn't get you awake. They talked to you and sang to you and wiped you with a cool cloth. You wouldn't wake up. We were all worried about you."

"That's ridiculous," I murmured, my eyes closing as if to erase the thought of such a thing. "They should have just asked me."

"Everyone just wanted you to be safe," Hunter told me, rubbing my arm. "The doctor will check you out and then we'll probably be on our way back to the rehab."

"Why would we go to the rehab?" I asked. "I want to go home."

Hunter gave me a light kiss and moved back from the bed, avoiding a long explanation that I wouldn't have understood anyway. I closed my eyes and eased my head back on the pillow. I could smell the beer on my husband's breath. Had we been out somewhere? Enjoying a summer evening together? Of course, we were. This must all be a dream.

Hunter called Ann after he tucked me safely in bed in my rehab room. I heard him say, "She is okay. There's really no point in your coming in until later in the morning.

Sorry this spoiled your one night out," he added, trying to console his daughter with his tone.

He told her to get some rest and he would call if there was anything new to report.

I felt him sit down on the edge of the bed. I opened my eyes to look at him. He looked awful. He was rubbing his forehead and murmuring to himself. I couldn't understand him.

I yawned lazily and pulled the blanket up to my chin. That's okay. I'll talk to him tomorrow.

"Where have you been?" I asked Brint accusingly, when he came to visit. I was in one of my terrible moods.

My son took my hand and squeezed it. He looked a little taken aback by my greeting.

"I'm sorry, Mom. I've been working a lot lately. This was the first chance I'd really had to make it in to see you."

I heard his words but I didn't believe him. He had a guilty look on his face.

I softened my tone after I saw the anxious way Brint rubbed his chin. Funny how that still struck a chord with me. Even when he was a little boy, when he needed to talk to me about something uncomfortable, he would rub his chin. My mood instantly changed.

"I just thought I might talk to you for awhile," he said hesitantly.

"Sure," I wanted to hug him and comfort him, but I couldn't. I didn't have the coordination left in my arms for a squeeze.

He started out slowly.

"Well, I just wanted to tell you about my awful night." He had my full attention. I was listening to him like a toddler would his favorite book.

"I kinda did something you wouldn't be very proud of." I could tell the words were painful for him to say. "In fact, I've Done quite a few things you wouldn't like lately," he confessed.

My sweet little Brint. He never did anything wrong. What was he talking about?

"I know you don't feel great and you have a lot of other worries, but I just think I would feel better if I told you some stuff." Brint gave a big sigh when he finished his sentence.

I nodded my head, giving him permission to continue.

"I've just been acting really stupid, lately," he said. "I've done some things that you would be mad at me for. And I probably shouldn't even be dumping this all on you, but if I don't tell you, it's just gonna eat at my insides."

Brint was rambling. He'd gotten that from his father. It always took him 10 or so sentences to even begin telling me what he didn't want to say. I waited for him to get to the point. He pulled up a chair and sat down.

"I'm just gonna tell you everything and then you can be as mad at me as you want," my son conceded. "I just feel like I'm keeping things from you since you've been sick. And I don't feel right about that. Even if you can't understand, I need you to hear my words."

Brint must be near the breaking point or he wouldn't be telling me anything, I thought. If Hunter or Ann or even Callie heard him dumping his problems on me, they would be appalled. Somewhere the mom in me understood perfectly.

"See, I've been partying a lot lately." My son squirmed like a little kid in his chair. "I know that sounds awful. There you are in a hospital bed and I'm out drinking and getting high."

His words would have startled me if my head was screwed on tightly. He was getting a break already.

"But I'm having a hard time dealing with all this about you, and everything. . ."

He paused to take a breath. I was hanging on every word.

"I'm not trying to blame you, but it's like, I just want to forget all this is happening. And partying does that for me. I can get with my friends and it's almost like you aren't even sick, like this whole summer never even happened. I can forget."

A tear in the corner of his eye caught my attention.

"I would just like to take all these bad days and put them in a box and blow them up—watch them explode and. . .forget. Forget! That's the only thing I can think of to fix all of this. I wish for it all the time. I pray for it. Then I curse it. I want to forget the long days and worries that come with me wherever I go. But I don't want to forget, because that probably means this whole thing is over, and there wasn't a happy ending."

His words touched me, even in my fragile state. My mom used to always tell my kids to put all their worries in a drawer and forget about them. That's what Brint was doing. Good boy!

"But when I forget, "he continued slowly, "I also forget how you used to be. It's getting harder and harder every day to remember the way you used to be. It's like, I have this picture in my mind of you, and it keeps changing. It goes from a picture of you standing in the kitchen all happy, making dinner and talking to us, to this sickening snapshot of you lying here in bed at this hospital...and you're slipping away from us a little more every day. All the great memories of you are fading."

The tear was down his cheek now, and another one started. Why was my poor little boy crying?

"It just doesn't seem like you are getting any better," he said, taking a deep breath. "And everyone's afraid to talk about it. No one will say the obvious truth. This horrible thing that you have is taking you over. Your looks, your speech, your whole you...it's being stolen away. And I'm mad at the doctors and nurses for not making you better. I'm mad at Dad because he won't face the truth. I'm mad at Ann because she thinks she's the only one losing you. I'm mad at Callie because she wants to be treated like an adult and she's only 14." He paused for just a second. "But I'm mad at you the most for not fighting this thing and getting better! It's your choice to get better or not, and...you're not. Don't you care about us? Can't you see what you are doing to our family?"

I couldn't grasp everything my son was saying, but some of it was sinking in. It was getting harder for him to remember the heart and soul of his mom, the one who used to care for him when he was little. He also could feel his worry turning into grief. The old me would have understood. It was like he was mourning the loss of me as he sat staring at me in this drab hospital gown. I was already gone, at least to him.

"Am I dying?" I asked, not even realizing the power it must have taken for Brint's thoughts to penetrate my mind.

Brint took my hand and put it up to his face, wet from tears. "I don't know, Mom. How long can you go on like this? How long can any of us?"

We sat and looked at one another for what seemed like a long time. He was so sad. Was it me doing that to him? The thoughts from just a moment ago had already left my brain. I looked at my son, waiting for him to speak. When he didn't, my thoughts changed course.

Am I dying? This time I asked myself. That was the biggest fear my kids always had. What could make him sadder than that? Nothing. That's what it has to be. I am dying.

How long till it happens? Am I facing months or years in this condition, fighting nurses to get out of bed, making crazy noises, seeing things that no one even listens to anymore? Every time I saw my husband or kids or my friends, they were all sad. I am doing that to them.

Ann walked into the room, noting our silence. It was obvious Brint had been crying.

"Everything in here okay?" she asked, panic taking over her facial expression as it had so many times before.

"Yeah," Brint nodded as he cleared his throat. "Me and Mom were just having a little talk."

Ann acknowledged my reply and pulled up a chair quietly. We all sat in silence for what seemed like hours. Brint spoke first.

"What's going to happen to her, Ann? Is this how it will always be?" He didn't want to hear the answer, but he did.

"I don't know," Ann said, tears filling her eyes. "They told Dad we needed to make some decisions."

I could tell Brint was trying to take in what his sister was saying. I was, as well.

"What kind of decisions? That's the type of thing they say when someone is not going to get better!" He stared at his sister. She didn't answer right away.

"Like what?" he finally asked, nastiness in his voice.

"They can't keep her here forever," Ann said, swallowing hard as the tears stung her eyes. "This is a rehab hospital, Brint. If a patient isn't improving, they've got to leave."

"What are we going to do?" he asked. His facial expression was totally clueless.

"Well, we could take her home or . . . ."

"Take her home?" Brint said, raising his voice. "We can't do that! It takes two nurses to even get her into the wheelchair! She can't walk from here to the door without falling on her face! She wears a diaper, for Heaven's sake! Who in the world thinks we can take her home?"

"I know, I know," Ann cried, her voice rising to match that of her brother's. "Do you want to hear what the other choice is? Do you want to know what else a caring, loving family could do for their mom?" She lowered her voice at the remote possibility I was listening. "They could put her in a nursing home! They could find some mental institution for crazy, demented old ladies and stick her in there. We could visit her on holidays and sit at home and knit slippers to keep her feet warm. What are we supposed to do, Brint? What do you think we should do? You have no idea what a full day in her life is like. All you do is hang out with your friends and stop in now and then to say hello. That's really easy for you. Do you even care what happens to her?"

The words, not meant for my feeble mind, conjured up visions of me tied in a bed at home, or a chilling image of me wrapped in sweaters, propped up in a chair, staring blankly into space at some drab nursing home. I wondered if Brint was thinking the same thing.

I could tell the resentment in his sister's voice made him angry. I knew my Brint. He wanted to scream at her.

"I'm doing my part too!" he replied in anger. "This isn't fun and games for any of us! Just because I'm not with her all the time doesn't mean I don't care!"

Brint glanced over his shoulder at me. My eyes were shut, but I was taking it all in. I was pleased to be hearing this exchange. It was a wonderful change from dead dogs and lunch menus. I almost wished I could join in.

My son continued with his rant. "Just because I'm not here with her every minute, also doesn't mean I'm not aware of the reality of things. I see what you see. I know how she's doing. I understand she's not getting better. But what is best for me may not be what's best for everyone else. You have your place here. Dad takes over when you need a break. I handle Callie and the dogs and I field the zillion phone calls we get each day on Mom's condition. And yes, I do hang out with friends occasionally. I find that a little more appealing than sitting at home alone, over-thinking things, wondering if today or tomorrow or next week is going to be the day Mom dies. Do you really want me to come in here and sit with you every day . . . because I can do that! If you think that's what I should be doing, then I will!"

Brint's voice was beginning to crack. His nerves had to be stretched thinner than he'd ever imagined possible. If he would have been little, he would have jumped on my lap and clung to me and hugged me until his fears disappeared.

Ann was crying. The explosion between the two of them had exhausted them both. They looked like limp rags in their seats, each probably wanting to take back what they had said, but glad for the chance to air things out.

Brint simply sat for a moment. I could tell he was contemplating his next move. In a movie, the brother would go over and hug his sister, reassure her everything would be fine. But this was reality. My son left without saying a word. Maybe later he could think through this again and get past Ann's hurtful words. For now, it was obvious they both needed time apart.

# Something's Wrong

❖❖❖

The next day brought relief from the heat spell we were having. I could feel the light breeze from the window. Although it was humid, the steady drizzle of rain throughout the day brought a coolness everyone welcomed. And yet, I was not having a good day. I seemed to be the focus of problems for everyone.

"Hey, Mom," Brint said cheerfully as he entered the room. He could tell by the solemn look on my face something was up. I didn't answer. I only motioned for him to come in.

"Hi Mom," Callie called. She was following her brother. When she got to me, her arms flew around my neck. "I need a hug."

"Sh-sh-sh!" I said, trying to put my finger to my mouth. My lack of coordination made that impossible, but they both knew what I meant.

"I have to tell you something." My voice was a whisper. My kids could hardly hear me over the noise in a busy hospital.

Brint and Callie came closer, waiting to hear my news.

"I'm getting another puppy," I said in words almost too soft to hear. Callie looked at me, a rare smile appearing on her face. Just the mere mention of a puppy again, no matter how deluded this idea was, sounded exciting to Callie.

"You are?" Callie asked. She had hopefulness in her voice.

"Sh-sh-sh!" I said again. "They'll hear you. If they hear you, they won't let it come."

"What's its name?" my daughter asked, playing along with the fantasy.

"I can't name him yet," I whispered in a somewhat irritated tone. "I have to see him before I name him."

Despite the oddness of it all, Callie had a look of relief in her eyes. Just being with me had to be enough for her right now. It didn't matter that my mind was full of nonsense and my tone was full of paranoia, I was still there, beside her, still being a mom.

Brint moved away from the bed. My imaginary world went on. I don't think he wanted to hear it. He wasn't the type to be calmed like Callie, with just the softness of my voice. He needed something real to hold on to.

Ann entered the room. She had been for a walk in the halls. She looked surprised to see them.

"I needed some time away from here," she said softly to Brint. She didn't appear to be harboring any resentment toward him over their last conversation

"About yesterday . . .," Brint said awkwardly.

"Forget it," she said. "We are both just tired and worried sick over this whole situation. I don't know how any of us talks civilly to anyone. It was good for us to both let off some steam."

Brint nodded. I could tell he was relieved their initial conversation for the day was over. They were both on the same team. I think my family felt that more now than ever.

"Callie was just pacing at home. She really needed to see Mom. I hope it's a good time for us to be here." I could hear his words. I looked to Ann for a reaction.

"Yeah, it's fine," Ann answered. "In Mom's mind today, there's a whole other world going on. Callie can tune into it for a while. When's Dad coming?"

"I don't know . . . haven't talked to him . . . probably after he takes care of the bills and stuff. I think he went grocery shopping."

"Shopping?" I repeated. My parroted response went unnoticed.

"Shoot!" Ann said, more to herself than to Brint. "I was going to do it tonight. I didn't want him to have to go."

"It gives him something to do," Brint told his sister, knowing he was right. "He's the picky one anyway. He can buy the stuff he'll eat."

I laughed in my mind. I could picture Hunter with a loaded shopping cart, going up and down the cookie aisle. Three fourths of his total order would be sweets. My thought made me hungry for some cookies.

Ann and Brint stood at the window, mentally listing the items for the grocery store. Callie and I were still talking quietly on and off about the new puppy.

I think it's time for 'The Young and the Restless' Ann sang as she turned on the TV. The song always relaxed me, no matter the state of my mind. I think it reminded me of summer days off at home with the kids. Sometimes I even fell asleep when it was on. I silenced everyone like I was watching it intently. Everything stopped—talking, noise, whatever. I'm sure that's what Ann was hoping for today. An early nap usually meant I would be more alert and easier to deal with in the afternoon.

The familiar sound of the theme song was Brint's signal to leave. He probably knew I would be safe with my soap opera family for a while. He was scheduled to work in an hour and still needed a shower.

"I'm staying to see the puppy," Callie said, still smiling at the fake news. Statements like this had become just another part of our crazy day. Strange actions, paranoia. . .they were normal now. I could feel the fight of my old self lessening within me. I was becoming content with being crazy. Occasional bouts of some semblance of reality hit me, but, for the most part, I lived in a world very different from anyone else. Could I be starting to like it?

The rest of my day brought nothing new. Therapy was pointless. I couldn't get even close to what they were asking of me. Rolling my neck on command was almost a joke. When I did try to do it, I must have pulled a muscle. I was in pain for the rest of the day.

I took a nap after supper and was plagued by the scariest of dreams. Two *Watchers* held me down while another one ran a razor blade across every part of my body. I cried for hours afterward. In reality, two nurses had been scrutinizing every part of my body, even inside my body cavities, for ticks. If I did indeed acquire Lyme disease recently, the tick might still be attached to me.

No amount of soothing from Ann would help. "They weren't trying to hurt you," she said, gently pulling my hair into a ponytail. "They had to check everywhere."

I was mad at Ann for allowing them to do it, and angry with Hunter for not being there for me. I held a grudge for hours.

My foul mood continued into the next day. Lunchtime was chaotic. The harder Ann tried to feed me, the more I resisted. By the time the lunch hour was over, I had thrown my utensils and spilled my lemonade all over the place. The nurses were worn down.

After they cleaned up the mess and changed my clothes, there was no time for therapy. The ladies put me safely in bed and left with me with Ann. My daughter would spend her afternoon making idle chit-chat and flipping channels on the TV. I made no valiant effort to get out of bed or even attempt to have a conversation. My spirit for life was literally dying. I could feel the hope slipping away with each passing hour. I was wasting the time of everyone around me.

By the time Dr. Hughes got back from his little vacation, I looked the worst yet. I was sitting in my wheelchair in the therapy room when he arrived. My mouth was open, I was drooling, my eyes were catatonic-like, and I seemed oblivious to everything around me.

"My God, she looks like she's stoned," Dr. Hughes uttered in disbelief. "I really thought she would be showing some positive signs by now. I stopped here on the way in the door. I haven't been down to my office to get her chart. Tell me how things were while I was gone."

Hunter gave him a brief rundown on what had been happening in the last few days. My condition worsened rather than improved like he had predicted. My tremors increased and it looked like I might be having some seizure activity again. I would become unresponsive for hours, being able to wince at pain, but unable to awaken if someone called me. My cognition had deteriorated as well. I was becoming more confused and almost appeared, at times, to be in a stupor. Since Dr. Hughes had been away, his partner made a decision in his absence.

"The other doctor increased the Depakote and took her off the Topomax," Hunter said, wondering if Dr.Hughes would have done the same.

"He said with her recent seizure activity, he assumed the Topamax wasn't doing its job. At that point, we were willing to try anything."

Dr. Hughes looked perplexed, but at the same time, Hunter could sense what Eve had told him about the doctor. The wheels were turning in his brilliant mind.

Hunter felt a stab of guilt pierce his heart at just the thought of Eve. Get used to it, he thought. That's a pain he would have to endure the rest of his life. Too many beers or not, there was no sane reasoning behind what he had done. Even though he hadn't slept with Eve, he'd made the mistake of wanting to. Hunter's sole focus now was on being there for me and doing everything possible to make me comfortable. He had given up on the idea of making me better.

"What are we going to do?" Ann quizzed Dr. Hughes, counting on him for an answer. "She's declining by the hour now."

"Hang in there," Dr. Hughes said. "I need some time." He wrote a few things down on a stray piece of paper and tucked it in his pocket. He left the therapy room and turned toward his office. Ann gave her dad a hopeful look. Both of them were convinced that if anyone was going to figure this out, it would be Dr. Hughes. But would he figure it out in time? By the looks of things today, I had very little left.

After my unsuccessful attempt at therapy, I was wheeled to my new placement at the nurse's station. They put me there any time a family member wasn't watching me. Ann left briefly to do a couple errands. It was obvious I was in the way. The women were busy bustling about the nurses' station—updating charts, checking on patients and conferring with doctors. One nurse, in particular, got my attention. She didn't mean to, but she sharply kicked my wheelchair as she scurried past me.

"Hey!" I yelled. The startled woman turned around and made her way to my side.

"I'm so sorry, Lisa. I bumped into you."

"Shut up, bitch!" I screamed, just inches from her face. My punch to her stomach came quickly. I smiled as I watched her double-over in pain.

I gritted my teeth and seethed—"You touch me again and I'll kill you!"

The scene was like out of a movie. Another nurse quickly stepped in. I grabbed her arm and dug my nails in. She squealed in pain. The left hook to her stomach caused even more ruckus.

"I hate you all!" I shouted.

I felt another body grab my chair and push me out of the work area. I was taken down the hall and into my room. I was still writhing in my wheelchair, trying to loosen the constraints.

"It's okay, Lisa," Dr. Hughes said, unbuckling the strap around my waist. He transferred me to the recliner and put the footrest up. I gave him a smile of gratitude.

He pulled up a chair and sat across from me. "You know, Lisa, everybody here is working really hard to make you comfortable. I think the nurses were just worried you were going to fall and they wouldn't see you."

I sighed. My mind was already past the incident. My eyes were fixed on the tv. I needed a break. Dr. Hughes turned it on and watched me calm down instantly.

Ann entered the room in a tizzy. She learned at the nurse's station what had happened. She apologized to the doctor as soon as she saw him.

"You know she didn't mean to hurt anyone," she added quickly. "My mom would be horrified if she realized what she did."

"I know," Dr. Hughes replied. "She should not have been placed in that situation."

Ann felt bad. She sat on the edge of my bed and looked at me. I was already asleep.

"I know she's getting hard to handle," Ann stated. "I think some of the nurses are even scared of her."

Dr. Hughes shook his head. "It's their job," he answered.

After a few seconds of silence, he stood up and moved to the door. "I'm going to have a nurse placed outside of her room round the clock. We can't take a chance of her falling out of her chair, or her bed during the night. We can keep her safe without the use of constraints. We just need to be more vigilant."

Ann watched as the doctor picked up my chart and wrote COMBATIVE at the top. He left the room to talk to the nurses down the hall. In a few minutes, a nurse appeared outside the door. She sat at a make-shift desk with a computer and a pile of paper work, with me in her vantage point. She couldn't have been happy with her new assignment.

My time at the nurse's station had exhausted me. I had expended so much energy worrying about the *Watchers*, I had none left to stay awake. This was becoming a bigger problem. As tired and listless as I was when I first came here, I was even more so now. After being awake for two to three hours, I needed a nap if I was expected to go to therapy or eat a meal. If I didn't get the rejuvenating naps, I either refused to complete the task or participated in such a hapless manner that I was excused from my responsibility.

I heard a nurse one day comparing my mind to Jell-O. Deep down, I knew she was right. And yet there was nothing I could do to restore it. I tried to pay attention at therapy and do what everyone asked, but so many things were just too hard for me. Every day was becoming longer and harder.

"Brint's here to see you," Hunter said, relieved to have something to divert my attention. He'd been trying to occupy me all day, like a parent does a little one. It wasn't easy. Fortunately, for them both, I'd just wakened from an hour's nap. I was as rejuvenated as I was going to get.

Brint! My heart did a little dance. One of my kids! I remember one of my kids!

"How are you?" I quizzed him as soon as he entered the room.

"I'm good, Mom," he said gently, giving me a hug.

"How are you?" he asked. It was a loaded question. The concerned party never knew what they were going to get—the Lisa who was mentally unstable, the Lisa who was not speaking because the *Watchers* were around, or the Lisa who reminded them of the woman she used to be.

I nodded at his question. I didn't know how to answer. The thought process to figure that out took more than one step. I didn't have that in me today.

"Have you seen Dylan lately?" I tried my best to act normal around my kids. This was a question I'd asked my son many times in his young life. Was my speech slurred? I felt like I was talking in an echo. My words vibrated in my head.

"Mom, Dylan moved away eight years ago."

Embarrassment should have engulfed me. It didn't.

"I know," I murmured, not really caring. I wonder what else I'd forgotten. My thoughts were so clouded. How did I come up with his friend's name at all? Wait, Brint must be the one mixed-up. He plays ball with Dylan in the backyard every day. They are in Pee Wee League together! What else was Brint confused about?

"What grade are you in?" I asked my son, not sure of the correct answer. I was asking random questions like my grandfather did in weeks before he died. The only difference was, he was in his eighties when he got dementia. I am only 51.

"I'm in college, Mom, remember?" His words were almost automatic, as if he expected the question.

"I know," I said quickly. "I meant, like, what grade are you in college?"

I should have been greatly embarrassed. But I wasn't. This was now my life. I spoke in riddles. I was getting used to it. Why couldn't the others around me do the same? Instead, they kept taking me down the hall to that big room, over and over, every day. They kept telling me to do tricks. Sometimes they would clap if I did them. But most times I just sat there until they took me back to my room.

I was a mess. I couldn't walk at all! I could barely talk! I couldn't even put those stupid little plastic thingies in the right spots to make the circle light up in therapy! Would I continue to deteriorate like this until I died?

Maybe I am extremely close to death now! That thought came into my head again. Maybe this is the end for me. A lot of people get crazy before they die. This must be what is happening to me!

I looked at my exhausted family. Despite my insanity, my heart ached for them. Maybe leaving this earth wouldn't be so hard. At least they would be relieved of the burden I had become.

"Lisa! Lisa! It's Michael, your nurse. I need for you to wake up. Come on, honey, open your eyes. I need to see you awake."

The annoying voice echoed in my ears.

"Lisa, honey, open those baby blues. Michael wants you to."

I couldn't tolerate the incessant whining any longer.

I squeezed my eyes shut tightly. I would outlast this guy. I was determined.

"Lisa, we don't want another trip to the hospital, do we?"

My mind, even in my confused state, recalled my previous visit to the ER due to being unresponsive. I opened one eye.

"That's a good girl," Michael said, fluffing my pillow. "How are you feeling?"

I tried to rub my eyes but my hands couldn't find them. I couldn't find my nose on my face! How am I feeling? You've got to be joking, Michael.

I mumbled an answer and tried to turn over, away from this intruder. But there was a tube sticking out of my arm. Michael could sense my curiosity.

"It's called a pic-line, Sweetie. It's a special place for us to give you your medicine. Let's not touch it. I know it's a little awkward but we don't really have a choice." Michael's reply did nothing to faze me. My hand instantly went to my arm. Fortunately, my poor coordination kept my fingers far away from the tube. My frustration mounted.

"Ann!" I announced, as my daughter came into the room. "I am . . ." I couldn't think of any more words.

"Mom, you're awake!" she whispered in relief. She gave me a huge hug then turned to Michael.

"How did you do it?" she asked the proud man standing nearby.

"He didn't do anything!" I sang out, glad to divert the attention back to me.

"You wouldn't wake up, Mom. Michael was giving you one last chance to come around before we loaded you up for the hospital. He's your hero today!"

"That's ridiculous!" I said, with a sour look on my face. "All you have to do is go 'click, click' and I will open my eyes. I'm a horse."

Ann barely smiled. The stress was wearing her down.

"Hey, guys!" I called, attempting to wave my arm in the air.

Ann and Michael turned around to see who had entered the room. There was no one there—except the television softly broadcasting a baseball game.

"Who are you talking to, Mom?"

"The guys," I said, glazed with exasperation. "How is everything going, guys?"

My conversation with the TV mounted to the wall was freaky. The sportscaster and ball players were in my room. I was sure of it! I talked on and off to them throughout the next hour.

A bug on the wall became my next fixation. I watched, stern-faced and mystified. What is that thing? Every time it moved a little, I gasped in confusion. Ann, not picking up on my tiny target, left the room. I was occupied by something, and that gave her a few minutes of freedom. When she came back, three of the *Watchers* were in my room.

"What's going on?" Ann asked, alarmed by the party of nurses.

"We're not sure," one of them said. "Your mom keeps ringing the call button."

Another added, "But when we get here, she won't talk to us. She just keeps staring at the wall."

"And she's acting like something is agitating her."

The group looked at Ann for answers.

When she got close enough to me, I grabbed my daughter's arm and pointed to the ceiling. Why did that dumb thumbtack up there keep moving around?

Ann spied the creature at the end of my gaze. She almost let out a laugh, but things weren't very humorous anymore. One of the nurses retrieved a broom from outside the hospital door and knocked the tiny insect off the ceiling. I acted like none of the last 15 minutes had ever happened.

I watched the parade of intruders going up and down the hall. I was happy none of them were coming in to see me. A nurse carrying a bouquet of flowers and four cards interrupted the next conversation my daughter and I were having.

"More flowers and cards from Dixie," I said, pleased with the tokens placed on my bed stand.

Ann did laugh at this. "Mom, not all flowers and cards are from Dixie. Other people are sending you get-well wishes too."

I looked right through my daughter as if she had never spoken. "I miss Dixie. It is so nice she sends me all this stuff."

In my mind, she was the only one who cared. I had known Dixie since we were kids. Now, I taught with her at the same school. The cards my kids had strung up through my room were actually from former students, relatives, and dear friends who cared very much. For some reason, Dixie was the only one who stuck with me.

"So, I hear congratulations are in order, Ann," the nurse said after lingering a bit.

Ann looked at the woman, wondering what she could possibly be talking about.

"I'm sorry," Ann said with a quizzical look. "I'm not sure I know what you are referring to."

"Your pregnancy," she smiled. "Your mom told everyone she saw this morning about your news. You must be so excited!"

I looked toward my daughter to see her reaction.

"Mommmmmmmmmm?" she sputtered in her 'what were you thinking?' mode.

"What?" I responded. "It's not a secret."

My daughter lowered her head, shaking it in disbelief. "Mom, you can't always have what you wish for. I don't even have a boyfriend. I think you're jumping the gun here."

The nurse turned a shade of pink that stood out against her platinum blonde hair.

"Oh, I'm so sorry," she whispered to Ann. "We sort of thought . . .."

Ann put her hand up to stop the woman from going any further. "It's okay. Really. If you could just kind of spread the word for me?"

"Sure," the young girl said, happy to be leaving the room. I watched her exit quickly. It was then I started to laugh.

"Mom," Ann let out in a chortle. "You can't make things up like this."

I started laughing . . . a good laugh—one I hadn't enjoyed in what seemed like forever. Ann joined in. We both laughed until tears rolled down our cheeks. It was the first sense of normalcy I'd felt since I'd gotten sick. If only I could bottle that feeling and bring it out when I wanted! I relished the moment until it faded to that dark place where all my "feel good" thoughts were sent to die. That place was becoming all too familiar.

Days passed by and I didn't fully realize the extent of my sickness or the hopelessness it brought to my family. Every day was the same. I got up, went to therapy, ate the meals, took my pills, and challenged the nurses. At night time, I often had fitful dreams. Most of the time, they centered around my family and who I used to be. Callie was always a baby in my dreams. She would cry and cry in my nightmare, but I could never get out of bed to get to her. Someone always held me back. My dreams were bittersweet, due to the fact that when I awakened, the normalcy was gone. My husband and kids were gone. It was just me and my crazy mind trying to figure out where I was and what was wrong.

"I need the trash can," I said to Callie one night.

"Are you sick?" she asked me in a worried tone.

"Umm, no!" I said rather harshly. My mind was all over the place. Random thoughts escaped my mouth. "All you do anymore is cry. . .cry. . .cry. . .cry. You're like a baby. You need to grow up. I can't take care of you for the rest of your life, you know."

My words were poison to Callie. No matter how much she was around me, she would never get used to my new sarcastic tone. She had no idea that, in my mind, she was still a little girl, dependent on me for everything. What I didn't know, was that I was the sole focus of her thoughts. The tears she shed all too often, were for me. Maybe I somehow sensed that. Maybe my recurring nightmares weren't that far off.

Callie swallowed tears and picked up the trash can. I shook my head and put my arms out for the container. The thoughts I'd had thirty seconds ago were gone. I felt a smile spread over my face as I saw the contents.

"I need that," I said pointing to the bottom.

Callie looked at me strangely then handed me the empty Cracker Jacks box.

"You already ate it all."

"I know," I said, trying to grasp the box. By this time, my small motor skills were practically non-existent. I couldn't hold the box without help.

"I need to be able to read it," I said impatiently. "Hold it up higher."

Callie followed my instructions and held the box up close to my face. She knew I couldn't read it, but she knew better than to argue.

"What are you looking for?" she asked, curious as to my actions.

"I'm tracking my calories," I said matter-of-factly. "Write this down—112597." Little did I know, I had just quoted Callie's birthdate. How I came up with it, I had no idea. There was definitely a little bit of the old Lisa in me still.

"Do you remember what the prize inside was?" Callie quizzed, forever hoping my memory would return.

"Inside what?" I asked. Callie mumbled something I couldn't hear. I could sense her disappointment in the air.

I put my head back on my pillow and sighed. I closed my eyes, hoping a daydream would envelop me. With any luck, I would be removed from this dreadful existence for even a short amount of time. Sometimes, when I shut my eyes, and began to relax, I would almost enter into another world. I often spoke out loud what I was visualizing or thinking. Today I talked of flowers and animals I may see outside. I rarely could remember what I was thinking about when I opened my eyes. But after those times, I appeared much more relaxed and lucid in my conversations. Perhaps that bit of a break was enough to regenerate a few new brain cells—ones which later on contributed to my sketchy piece of mind.

My therapy was cancelled again the next day due to my much-worsening condition. I wasn't able to respond to anything asked of me. From minute to minute, it was hard to tell if I even realized where I was or if I recognized my family around me. My morning consisted of dumping my oatmeal, arguing with a nurse who wouldn't let me out of bed, and yelling at my husband for not caring about me. By noon, everyone involved had about had it with me. Hunter wasn't surprised when the director of the hospital soon showed up.

"Mr. Church, I understand your wife's not having a very good day."

Hunter nodded, unable to contradict her. "I guess she laid into a couple nurses."

That was putting it politely. I had lashed out verbally at anyone near me all morning. By afternoon, I was punching and kicking. Fortunately, my aim was so off, I hadn't really hurt anyone. But I was in a dark mood. Everyone, including my family, knew I was at my most difficult today for some reason.

"I know this has been so hard on you and your family. We all want what's best for your wife." She paused, allowing the words to sink into Hunter's muddled mind. He knew it would be bad news.

"We are a therapeutic hospital. A rehabilitative facility such as ours can only keep patients who are improving, actually responding to the therapy we have to offer. I think you would have to agree that the help we've been providing Lisa just isn't enough. In fact, her therapy at this point is almost nonexistent."

"But Dr. Hughes is actively working on her case. He strongly believes that she is going to get better!" Hunter pleaded.

"Well, this is strictly from the hospital's guidelines. By all means, your wife could still see Dr. Hughes as an outpatient."

Hunter could barely keep himself from fleeing the room.

"I have a short list here of facilities in the area who take patients with brain disorders. They have a special wing for people suffering from dementia or Alzheimer's. They are terrific at what they do. We just feel Lisa would be so much more comfortable in a setting where she is treated by staff trained exclusively for patients with dementia."

If she was waiting for Hunter to respond, she would only hear the deafening silence in the room. He took the paper and stared at it. The words looked foreign to him. Hunter read the list of nursing homes, unable to fathom placing me in such a center. And yet, the advice of the director made sense. It was obvious I was not responding to therapies. This move had been only a matter of time.

"Please feel free to call or visit these places. I've already been in touch so they will know the scenario beforehand." She gave Hunter's shoulder a sympathetic pat and turned to leave the room.

"How long do I have?" he called out, finally finding his voice.

"Just a few days."

Pause.

"I'm sorry, Mr. Church."

"I know," he said. "I know." He watched her walk away, taking with her the only hope he had. Without Dr. Hughes constantly checking in on me, and the care of the staff at this rehab, he was sure I would never make it. I would just wither away to nothing and be forgotten. He turned around and just looked at me. My head was back on my pillow, but I was far from asleep. My blue eyes were wide open, staring at the ceiling. He walked over to me and took my hand. He squeezed it softly and said my name. In the movies, this would have been the scene where I would blink my eyes, look at my husband, and come out of my stupor. But this wasn't the movies. And I didn't even know he was there.

Hunter was going crazy himself. Why couldn't anyone figure out what was wrong with his wife? For the first time, he could feel anger growing inside of him... not at God or the doctors or fate... but at me—just as Brint had. Why was I doing this to them? Why didn't I fight harder to come out of this? Why couldn't I just look at him, so he could find the "old me"—the girl he used to laugh and argue with, hold in his arms and make everything better? How could I just lie there, knowing my kids and mom and rest of my family were worried sick over me? Couldn't my will to live be stronger than this monster that was trying to destroy me? Would I actually let it succeed? It was too much for any spouse to comprehend.

The door opened. Hunter turned around and saw Ann. The look on her face was exactly how he felt.

"We are," Hunter said to her, "in need of a miracle."

By the morning of my birthday, August 1, I had been in the hospital for 26 straight days. Time was marching on.

"Happy Birthday!" Ann chimed as she entered my room at 7:00 a.m. I'd already been up for an hour, but the day's significance never entered my mind. For some weird reason, I knew "thank you" was an appropriate response.

"I brought you some presents!" my daughter sang, holding up a bag of goodies.

I felt like a little kid. The excitement of what Ann said made me tingle with pleasure. It probably seemed strange to my daughter to see me this anxious for presents. I had always been one of those people who was hard to buy for. When I opened a gift from someone, I typically feigned my true response.

Seeing me happy about the actual holiday was also unique. I'd stopped counting birthdays long ago, about the same time I got my first wrinkle. But today, for some reason, in that shallow brain that I had left, I felt like this one was special. Was it because it was my last? I was too unstable to entertain the thought.

"Give me, give me!" I said with delight. "I'm so excited!" My mood fit the day.

She quickly handed me an oddly shaped package and helped me unwrap it.

"Just what I've always wanted!" I squealed, holding the object close to my face. My tunnel vision had become so bad I couldn't make out an object unless it was squarely in front of me.

Ann looked pleased as punch. "It's a cup with a straw already attached. Do you like it?"

"I love it! How did you know I always wanted one of these?"

"Oh, I just made a lucky guess. We'll practice using it in a little bit. Maybe you'll be able to hold it all by yourself."

Rather than be offended by the challenge, I reveled in it. "Of course I will!" I said proudly. "You can help me!"

My favorite therapist, Robin, walked in the room and smiled. "I heard you have a birthday today, Lisa!"

I was beaming with happiness. "Yes, come here my little Robin," I said in a playful tone. I patted the edge of my bed, encouraging her to sit.

"I love the present you got me!" I pointed to the cup Ann had purchased for me. Poor girl! It was probably the first time she saw me truly impressed with a gift, and now she didn't even get credit for it.

"Your daughter got that for you," Robin said, giving Ann a wink. "It's nice."

"No, you got it for me. Thank you very, very, very much!" I gave Robin a hug before she scurried back to work.

"What else do you have for me?" I asked my daughter. My eagerness was over the top. "Open these," she said, handing me another wrapped gift.

I fumbled with the paper and finally turned the package over to Ann for help. When I saw the contents, I was just as excited as when I saw my cup.

"Oh my gosh!" I whispered, acting like she'd handed me a check for a thousand dollars. "These are great!" I couldn't think of the name for them but I knew what to do with them. I unfolded the arms and tried to put the sunglasses on my face. Ann put them on me as she would on a child. My hands wouldn't allow me to do it myself.

"How do I look?"

Ann laughed and gave me a thumbs-up. "You look wonderful! They'll be great for when I take you for your walks outside here."

"I love them!" I tried to get up and walk to the mirror. Ann stopped me as she had hundreds of other times this summer.

"You have one more to open," she interjected, handing me another gift. She had already started to open it so I ripped the rest of the paper off with ease.

"It's a puppy!" I whispered, shocked at what I was holding. I couldn't believe my daughter had actually gotten me a puppy!

I grabbed the stuffed animal and hugged it with a vengeance reserved only for little children in my prior sane life. I rocked it and talked to it like it was the newest member of our family. If I had been 6 years old, this would have been endearing. At 52, it was just plain sad.

When the door to my room opened, I grabbed the dog and instinctively hid it under blankets. I prayed no one would take it from me.

"They won't let me keep it!" I whispered in sheer panic. "We have to hide! We have to hide!"

Ann wanted to laugh . . . or cry. My delusions these last few weeks became the norm. "Did you see that?" I would say with fear in my eyes. "Do you see that man looking at us?" Ann would just shake her head and change the subject. "Don't look over there!" I said one day. "Those people know we are here and they are talking about us." Ann assured me they were just nurses doing their jobs. I looked at her, frightened and trembling, telling her not to trust them. She even had to put something over the window in the door, as they had at the last hospital, to keep me placated. No reassurance from anyone would alleviate my fear. Ann mimicked, in a soothing tone, niceties that I had used with her when she was young and frightened. She did her best to keep me calm.

Callie and Brint came in next, with big smiles on their faces. Were they laughing at me? Did they somehow find out about the puppy already? Where were my presents? Wasn't this my birthday?

"I made you a cake," Callie said proudly, putting the lopsided object on my bed tray. "I know you can't eat it, but it's the first layer cake I've ever made without you helping. Isn't it great?" I know I saw a tear in my daughter's eye. I had no idea how hard this day was for her.

I smiled at the sight and swiped my finger at it, trying to reach the frosting. I looked pathetic, not even getting within six inches of my target. Ann got a spoon and gave me a small bite. My diet was so limited—no sweets, no dairy, no wheat, no beef . . . only fruits and vegetables until they figured out what was wrong with me. But, hey, it was my birthday. My pleasures in life now consisted of being able to sleep as long as I wanted, and getting to see my kids, but even that one was fading. I forgot about the cake the second it was whisked away. The old me would have had a piece for breakfast, lunch and supper since I adored sweets.

The room cleared out except for Callie. She stood and looked at me like I was a stranger. Her smile was there, but I knew it was only out of courtesy.

There was an uncomfortable silence between us that had never been there before. What could she say to me? I had once been her best friend, now we were almost strangers.

A nurse entered the room. I screamed at her to get out and raised a fist to her.

"Mom," Callie said in surprise, "she's just checking on you."

My outburst had scared my daughter. My actions were getting more violent each day. She'd seen me in altercations with the staff more than once. If only I could make her see I was fighting off the *Watchers* to protect my family.

I tucked my puppy down further under the covers, hiding it until the nurse left the room. If that's what it took to keep this dog, so be it, I thought. It was my birthday. I finally have my very own dog. Nothing would interfere.

Despite my good spirits at the onset, my day proved to be long for everyone involved. Eating breakfast seemed to take forever. Ann fed me as usual. Her hopes that my hands would stop shaking vanished. I trembled to the point where even my large motor skills were affected. Holding anything fragile was out of the question. And therapy? It had become almost a moot point.

I wasn't fooling anyone. This was just a place to house me—a temporary stop on my way to a nursing home. There, someone could relieve Ann. She could get her life back. She could be free of obligations. My husband could limit his visits as well, giving him time to focus on being a single parent. My kids would muddle through life with a burden on their shoulders. I would be a constant concern. My grandchildren's memories, if I made it that far, would be of a woman in a hospital bed, oblivious to her surroundings and unable to recognize her offspring. It was fortunate that I didn't comprehend these realities. Dealing with them, had I been alert, would have broken my heart.

"Katie is on the phone for you, Mom. She wants to tell you happy birthday." Ann handed me her cell phone and watched for my response. I put the object up to my ear like it was a foreign object I'd never seen before. I was surprised when I heard a voice on the other end.

"Go!" I said, not even knowing to whom I was speaking. I nodded with acknowledgment at the voice but I didn't know who this Katie person was. And why was she wishing me a happy birthday? It wasn't my birthday!

The conversation was sad. It was obvious Katie had asked me my age. The answers I gave her ranged from my birth date and my phone number, to my house number and my room number at school—all jumbled together. I could hear the lady on the other end begin to cry. I handed the phone back to my daughter and leaned back in my bed, oblivious to all whom I affected.

For some strange reason, during the afternoon, I began to get more confused. I couldn't remember how to move my mouth, nor could I recognize faces. I could feel myself sinking into an abyss. The everyday world moved on, but I was stuck in a black hole. I couldn't get out. I didn't even want to. This was going to be the end for me. I could feel it.

I could sense my family around me, perhaps calling my name softly, or patting my hand. But it was no use. I couldn't get back to them. I had finally reached the end of the journey, this nightmare, this hell that I put everyone through. It had come to an end.

I was semi-conscious, languishing in a hospital bed in the middle of my room. I was a mound of rubble, a useless mass taking up space. I could accept no attention or affection, nor could I offer it to others. My mind was blank. I had finally turned the tide. . .unfortunately in the wrong direction. I was ready to be dismissed from everything around me. The sensation was frightening, yet soothing. There had to be an end.

❖❖❖

Hunter entered my room about 4:30 p.m.

"I'm glad Callie came in this morning," I heard Ann say to her dad. "Mom was much better then. We gave her a couple of presents. She talked and laughed with us. But she started to get very paranoid again, a lot like she was in Ohio. I can't believe she's gotten this much worse since this morning."

At that moment, Dr. Hughes stepped in the room. The smile on his face didn't make sense. Couldn't he see how drastically I had declined in such a short period of time? Hunter and Ann waited for him to talk.

"I have a couple of things I want to do here," Dr. Hughes said, quite upbeat. "We discussed the possibility of Lyme disease a few days ago. Even though Lisa has had no miraculous recovery after the first few days on the antibiotic, that is not a sign that she isn't infected with Lyme. Like most things, antibiotics take a while to work. And remember, that's one medicine that won't hurt her if I'm wrong. We have to remember there was something slowly tearing her body down for months now, possibly years. We have to address that, along with the fact something else could be causing her dementia." He paused to let my husband and daughter digest everything he was saying.

"While I was away, her Depakote dosage got increased when the Topamax didn't seem to be working. With such a small change making her decline so rapidly, that made us think the problem has to be metabolic—the whole range of biochemical processes that occur within a person. If she reacted so drastically to changes in her medications, the cause of the symptoms has to be outside her body to cause this harm. She was put on Depakote the end of May. Didn't her problems significantly increase right after that?"

Hunter and Ann looked at each other and nodded, trying to comprehend everything. Could this be good news?

"So," he concluded, "my colleagues and I discussed taking her off the Depakote totally. We're not even weaning her off slowly. It is our guess that this is the root of the dementia problem. The Depakote is probably the reason her ammonia level increased as well. Her reaction to the Depakote is wreaking havoc all through her. We should see her greatly improve, simply by stopping this drug. I don't want her to have the Topamax either. Lisa actually could have been negatively reacting to it over the years like she has suspected. I'm putting her on a drug called Keppra to prevent the seizures. Despite her sensitivity to a lot of medicines, I think she will do well on this one.

"We can take care of the Lyme issues as they come." The doctor smiled and continued, looking at each one of us. "I say—plan the birthday party. Things are looking up!"

"Could it really be that easy?" Ann asked, more to herself than anyone else.

Hunter simply stood in a daze, trying to process the optimistic words he'd heard. I'm sure neither one was having an easy time believing there was actually a chance I could get any better. It had been too long. There was too much damage to my brain.

At this point, my family needed more than a prediction. They needed a promise. They needed some proof. Dr. Hughes left the room with a smile on his face. Only time would tell.

The next day brought no changes. I tried to go through the motions like every other day, but the routine was now more of a challenge than ever. Therapy was discontinued. My interest in meals was gone. I was being spoon-fed like an old lady, sitting motionless except for the strain to swallow every few bites. As crazy as I was, even I could sense the tension in the air. My night had been filled with terror and madness. I woke up every few hours, thrashing and yelling, trying to get out of the bed that kept me safe. The nurses were growing even more fearful of me. I would kick, hit and punch any time I didn't get my way.

And my family. . .they kept looking at me like they expected something. I felt no different than the day before. Each day was a rerun. The reruns in the hospital were now memories. Did I choose to forget things these days or was I incapable of any worthy functions? My thoughts were exhausting and filled with jumbled nonsense. For some odd reason, 'your brain is fried' kept repeating itself in my head. Had someone recently told me that? Had the *Watchers* etched that phrase in my mind when I wasn't looking? Is that what I was supposed to believe?

That night, when my husband was getting me ready for bed, I noticed for the first time in months the tender way he treated me. He brushed my teeth, washed my face, and changed me into my nightgown. All the while he talked softly to me, telling me soothing moments from the day. I could see the strain and worry on his face, but he didn't let on about any concerns. He kissed me good night, told me he loved me, and covered me up. He sat down in the recliner beside my bed and just looked at me. I wanted to tell him something, but I didn't know what. More importantly, I didn't know how. My mouth kept moving to speak but no words came out. But rather than feeling fear or paranoia, I felt a calm relief sweep over me. I shut my eyes and let the feeling sink in. I drifted off to sleep feeling loved, cared for, and a little more in tune with reality.

My sleep that night was different too. My dreams weren't of me trying to get out of bed to rescue a crying baby. They weren't about someone trying to keep me away from my children. They were about my life . . . as it used to be. I saw my children at different ages. I saw my home in the country. I saw Lisa Church, the way I used to be. It was all so relaxing and peaceful.

That next morning, I awoke early. I was kind of on my own schedule. It had been decided for my last few days here to let me sleep-in in the mornings. Having me get up at 7 a.m. to fight with the nurses and refuse my breakfast was productive for no one. On nights I slept, it was usually 9:00 before I started to stir.

Not even thinking about what time it was, I pulled back the covers and unclipped the alarm attached to me. I got out of bed. I stepped to the floor, a little wobbly at first, but my atrophied legs were able to support me. I took the eight steps or so to the restroom and picked up my toothbrush. Why am I so shaky, I wondered. I fumbled a little getting the lid off the toothpaste. Putting the gel on the toothbrush was a bit of a challenge as well, but I managed to do it. I leaned into the sink and moved the brush around my mouth. I felt a strangeness at what I was doing, but I wasn't sure why. I was just brushing my teeth! I awkwardly turned off the water and grabbed a towel off the rack. I had toothpaste all around my mouth. A little messy today, I noted. I dabbed my mouth dry and returned the towel to its spot.

"Mom!"

My daughter's voice startled me. I turned around quickly to see who it was. I lost my balance, but just for a second. Somehow I managed to stay upright.

"Ann!" I gasped, putting my hand to my heart. "You scared me!"

My daughter just stood there, her jaw to the floor. She appeared even more startled than me.

"You're out of bed!" she exclaimed, still trying to grasp what she was seeing.

I laughed slightly at her comment. "It is morning, you know."

My daughter moved in closer as if she needed to touch me to confirm what she was seeing.

"What's the matter?" I asked, perplexed at her puzzled look.

Tears came to her eyes as she reached out to me. I put out my arms, confused as to why she was crying.

"What's the matter?" I asked again, this time a little worried.

"How did you get out of bed?" she whispered, still squeezing me tight.

"I just did," I answered, taking a step back to look at her once again.

"Do the nurses know?" Tears kept streaming down her cheeks.

"I guess not. I haven't seen any of them. "Why?"

"Come on, Mom, let's get you back into bed."

"I'm not going back to bed," I replied quickly. "I just got up!"

Ann shook her head, apparently not believing what I said.

"Okay," she laughed. "How about we sit you in this chair for now?"

I nodded in agreement and took her outstretched hand to guide me there.

"I don't know why I'm so shaky today," I said, once again referring to the trembling of my hands. "I actually feel a little weak as well. Let me think about what I did yesterday. Maybe my workout was a little too harsh on my body."

Ann was the one shaking this time. Her hand quivered in mine as she put the footrest up on the recliner to make me more comfortable.

"I have to call Dad," she said quickly, more to herself than to me.

"Tell him I said hello," I said sincerely. "It feels like I haven't seen him in. . .forever."

Ann's phone was out of her pocket in a flash. She pressed the numbers then raised her trembling hand to her ear.

"You have to come quick," I heard her say. "No, nothing's wrong . . . nothing's wrong . . . it's Mom. When I walked in the room she was out of bed and brushing her teeth by herself!"

I shook my head at her words. Wow, brushing my teeth by myself—since when was that an accomplishment in our family?

"Dad will be here soon!" she said with excitement.

"Great!" I said. "Hey, let's go for a walk." I fumbled with the footrest, trying to get it back down.

"Whoa!" my daughter chuckled. "We can go for a walk but you better let me push you in the wheelchair."

"Seriously?"

"Well, then we can go for a walk outside. How would that be?" Ann's suggestion made me smile. I didn't know it was a diversion tactic. She had grown quite proficient at those over the summer.

"Wonderful," I responded, quite receptive to the news. "Do I have to get dressed first?"

"No way!" My daughter's answer was more of a command. "I want everyone to see you the way you are!"

This time I chuckled. "I don't even have my makeup on! But then, who's going to see us anyway?"

My laissez faire attitude was already resurfacing. I allowed Ann to help me up from the recliner and into a nearby wheelchair. Although I was fragile, I was gung-ho compared to my last several weeks.

I adjusted myself to a comfort level that suited Ann. She clicked off the brakes on the chair and maneuvered me out of the room. We buzzed through the hall and out the nearest door. It was almost as if she didn't want me to be seen yet.

I welcomed the outdoors like a long-lost friend. Everything seemed so vibrant.

"What beautiful asters," I commented as we passed a patch of wildflowers that actually did include asters. "The purple in them is almost a lavender color."

Ann acknowledged my statement and waited for more.

"Look at that groundhog standing up over there!" I blurted out, hoping my daughter would see it before it crouched too low behind the tall grass. "And there's a goldfinch! I don't know when the last time was that I saw one of those!" I began to note everything—flowers, trees, wildlife, the cool morning breeze. It was like I was seeing and feeling things for the first time. I was actually entertaining myself as well as Ann.

"Look at that butterfly!" I mused, pointing toward some milkweed in bloom. "Its colors are magnificent!"

"You can see that butterfly?" Ann retorted.

"Of course," I said. "It's right there."

"It's just that you were having some problems with your eyes for a while. I'm so happy you're doing better." From what she could tell, my vision was back to normal.

"Oh," I said in a satisfied voice. "I can see fine now."

Ann smiled. "Do you remember the names of these flowers?" she asked as we passed a cluster of daisies.

"Duh!" I answered, making her burst into laughter. I took the next minute or so to spew out nouns—names of every wildflower and animal I saw.

"You haven't missed a one!" Ann beamed proudly. "You're back, Mom. You're really back!

My husband was waiting for us when we got back to the room. One look at me confirmed what Ann had told him earlier.

"Hey," I said. "Sorry to keep you waiting. We were checking out all the wildflowers outside."

I will never forget the look on his face when he first saw me. To have gotten back the love of his life, practically overnight . . . to know that I was actually okay—speaking, moving, remembering. . . it was surreal. Our eyes caught for the briefest moment. But our hearts locked for eternity. He walked to my chair and took me in his arms. Our embrace had everything a love story was made of . . . commitment, loyalty, faith, strength. Hunter never gave up, despite his close call to indiscretion with Eve and challenges he faced with me every day.

"I love you," he said, the back of his hand gently caressing my cheek. "I'm so glad you came back to us."

I gave him a warm smile in return. "I love you too."

"Can you believe this?" Ann said, bursting with excitement. "I got here this morning and she was in the bathroom by herself! She was standing there, on her own, brushing her teeth!"

"Okay," I finally said. "So what is the big deal with me brushing my teeth?" My mind was racing, trying to piece the details of this situation together. Up until this moment, I hadn't questioned where I was or why. I had just accepted it.

"It's amazing, Mom, because you couldn't even walk at this time yesterday. Your speech was slurred, your energy was zapped, you could hardly remember anything!"

I heard Ann's words, but trying to absorb them was a different story. Couldn't walk? Slurred speech?

"Where am I?" I finally asked, becoming more and more aware of my surroundings. "Why am I here?"

I guess the best way to describe my mindset from the moment I woke up that morning till that moment is that I was living totally as if I had just awakened from a dream. The world around me was almost electric. The lights were brighter, the sounds were clearer, the images crisp and new to me. When I saw a flower, it was like the most beautiful flower in the world, until I saw the next one. It felt like I was coming alive, regaining my sight, and hearing beautiful, eloquent sounds for the first time. Taking it all in was almost overwhelming. I had been too busy soaking up the world to think about the details. Nothing seemed real. Everything seemed real.

"You are at a rehab hospital," my husband answered gingerly, unsure yet of my stability.

"Why?" I asked, blown away by what he said. "Was I in an accident or something? Wait! Where are the kids? Is everyone okay?"

"They're fine. I promise," Hunter answered quickly.

"Okay," I said, taking for granted what he told me. My brain was still foggy, my thinking a little unclear.

Hunter continued. "You had a reaction to a medicine that you were put on to stop seizures. That's mainly why you're here. The doctor also thinks you might have Lyme disease. That's why your memory was getting bad and you were having trouble walking."

I looked at him in disbelief. "How long have I been here?" I asked him, not anticipating what he'd say.

"Over a month."

I shut my eyes, trying my best to comprehend what he said. "I've been here that long?"

"Yeah, you've been pretty sick."

"Did you think I might. . .die?" I asked, looking over to Ann. I was horrified at the thought of putting them all through this.

Ann nodded her head and fought back tears. "We didn't know, but I think in our hearts, we always knew you'd come back to us."

I reached over and gave my daughter a tight squeeze. "I'm so sorry," I whispered. "It must have been awful."

"It's okay," she whispered, still getting used to the idea that her mom would be all right. "You're here now, and getting better, and that's all that counts."

I sat back to allow all this information to register. "Did you guys ever come to visit me?"

Hunter and Ann looked at one another, unable to hold their laughter in. I couldn't imagine what was so funny.

"Oh, we visited you," Ann answered. "You had someone with you from sun-up to sun-down."

I laughed to relieve some of my own tension. It was strange, waking up in a hospital and learning that you had been absent from the rest of the world for more than a month. I was so happy to hear that my family had stuck by me through all this.

"Do Brint and Callie know I'm feeling better?" I asked, anxious to see my other two children.

"Not yet," Hunter said, "but I will text them, and you can surprise them yourself when they get here. Callie is probably at the park with Rose by now, and Brint may be working. They will be here today for sure!"

"Right now, I'll bet there are some nurses and doctors who will enjoy seeing you like this," Ann added as she walked to the door. "I'll go leave word at the nurse's station for them to stop down."

I smiled. I couldn't wait to meet them.

Ann returned from the hallway with three nurses behind her. It was obvious she hadn't told them yet. All three stood in the doorway, mouths open, staring at what they saw.

"He did it," one said, shaking her head in disbelief. "Dr. Hughes said he was going to make you better."

"He wasn't kidding," another one added. "I can't believe what I'm seeing."

"Dr. Hughes is gonna freak!" the third nurse said.

In a wonderful burst of chaos, the women showered us with a hundred questions—all on how this could be possible. It was funny. Ann and Hunter talked to them like they were old friends. But I felt as if I had never seen these women before in my life. I sat back and enjoyed all the chatter. The nurses must have been a pretty caring bunch for such a display of happiness. I immediately warmed to them, sensing their commitment and care they most assuredly had given me.

One left the room to tell the others. Before I knew it, I had a circle of friends I'd never met standing around me. One after the other, they stayed a few minutes then left to tell someone else. There were phone calls made to their family and friends, telling of the "miracle" at their workplace. Breakfast was brought to my room by one of the cafeteria workers, wanting to see for herself that Lisa Church was actually better. They watched in awe as I held a fork in my hand, ready to take on a pancake and a few slices of banana. When I actually made it to my mouth, with a little help from Ann, they responded with a round of applause. I blushed at their attention and put my fork down. I was happy they were happy. I was glad to be alive!

Ann went with me to the shower room to get me freshened up and dressed in everyday clothes. Although I was weak, I stood in the shower alone, my daughter only a few inches away to grab me if I became unsteady. I made it through, even washing my hair for this special occasion. Ann helped me dress in real clothes, babbling the whole time about the drab hospital gown and the weather and how nice the nurses were here at the hospital. I didn't know she was making every effort to keep my thoughts on the here and now. The terrible happenings from the last month or so could be explained later. Right now, she just wanted to revel in the happiness of this moment.

When we returned to my room, Hunter was standing near the window, talking with a gentleman I didn't know. He was dressed neatly and professionally, with a white coat on. I wasn't sure who he could be. But when I entered the room, the look of pride in his eyes let me know he was someone special.

"Dr. Hughes?" I said, extending my hand. I'd heard his name mentioned dozens of times in the short amount of time I'd been up.

He smiled and shook his head in disbelief. It was as if he was meeting me for the first time. To me, he was. He took my hand and squeezed, unable to draw his gaze away from me. I felt exactly the same way. We had a connection that I couldn't yet understand.

"I have a lot of questions for you," I said softly. His smile let me know he would be all too happy to answer every one of them. He promised a complete explanation in a little while. But right now, he needed to get my vital signs and make sure all my parts were working. After all, reawakening like this had to be somewhat of a shock to my system. He took my blood pressure and pulse and performed a few other little tests to confirm I was in workable order. He left the room, promising to be back later. He also canceled any therapy sessions for the morning. He thought I deserved a little downtime with my family.

While I had been showering, Hunter made, what seemed to him a thousand phone calls. He must have told my story of revival a hundred times, but he didn't mind. It had a happy ending. Hopefully, I just needed some time to rest and build up stamina.

"I called Rose to let her know you're feeling better," Hunter said, giving me a kiss on the cheek. "We're going to surprise Callie, though. I told Rose to keep it a secret. She offered to end their park adventure early and come right over. But Callie seemed to be enjoying herself, so I told her to let them go a little longer."

That suited me fine. As much as I couldn't wait to see my family, I also was tired. Taking my shower thoroughly exhausted me. There was enough going on right now. Perhaps later, I would get to spend my quieter moments with Callie. I smiled, picturing her in her blue jeans and favorite shirt. I drifted into a nap with a smile on my face.

I woke up in an hour as lunch was being placed in front of me. I looked around to remind myself of what was happening. Ann and Hunter were at my bedside, praying I would again wake up coherent and alert. I had.

"Aren't Brint and Callie here yet?" Their names rolled off my tongue hesitantly, but I had said them, nevertheless; a remarkable improvement from a day ago.

"A little bit later," Hunter said, unable to keep the smile off his face.

"Callie is at the park with Rose and Brint had to work. They'll be here as soon as they can." He repeated the words to me out of habit. Up until now, everything had to be told to me numerous times for merely the essence to sink in. His words warmed my heart. He could say them a hundred times, I didn't care. I was still getting bits and pieces of how things had been for me the last several weeks. But as long as I had my family around me, I knew the days ahead would be fine.

"Callie is going to go crazy when she sees you," Hunter said, anticipating the moment almost as much as I was.

I smiled. "Is she having a nice summer?"

Clearly my way of thinking was focused on a typical summer day with my kids—unlike what they were experiencing this summer. I had no idea, yet, the extent of my illness and the effect it had had on all of them. Ann felt she should broach the subject a little before her brother and sister got here.

"Callie has been so worried about you, Mom. She will be elated that you have come back to us."

I kept hearing "you have come back." "Was I dead?" I finally asked, looking to Hunter for an answer.

"No," he said, "but you've been pretty sick. We weren't sure there, for a while, if you were going to make it."

Tears came to my eyes. I swallowed hard and took a deep breath.

"I'm sorry." That was all I could muster right now. If I dug any further into the situation, I may have ruined the jubilant mood.

I ate my lunch with Ann's help. I still didn't have the motor control that it took to get a fork into the food, then into my mouth efficiently. It was going to take some time to get my body back in 100 percent working order. I was weak and my thinking was still somewhat cloudy. I needed to take one day at a time, they said, and give myself a chance to heal. I didn't realize this right away, but as time went on, it became apparent. I did not wake up this morning all fixed and ready to go. I had lots of work ahead. But, oh. . . what an improvement!

Dr. Hughes favored me going to therapy in the afternoon, so Ann cheerfully took me down the hall to the gym. The therapists had all heard the news, but were waiting to see for themselves the progress I'd made, almost overnight. Robin, whom I didn't remember ever meeting, gave me a big hug when she saw me. She had tears in her eyes.

"I feel kind of silly," I said to this young girl. "You people here all seem to know me so well. I don't even remember seeing you before. It's kind of unfair."

Robin gave me a sympathetic look. "I guess it is kind of weird for you. Don't worry, though, you will come to know me very well in the next several days. I promise you that."

Ann laughed. "Oh yeah, Mom, she will put you through the wringer! You'll never forget her."

I tried to laugh it off and concentrate on the small tasks. Every time I felt a bit defeated, I thought of Callie and Brint. I couldn't wait to see them. That thought kept me going!

I didn't have to wait too long. By the time I got back to my room, Callie was sitting on the side of my bed waiting. I watched the relief replace the stress on her face. "Mom!" she cried, jumping off the bed and down to my level in the wheelchair. "I thought something terrible had happened! I got here and your bed was empty and no one would tell me where you were!"

She still didn't realize the transformation that had taken place. I stood up slowly from the wheelchair. The smile I'd been waiting for appeared.

"She's getting better!" Ann said with a new confidence. "Mom is really getting better!"

Tears came to Callie as she stood back and looked at me.

"I'm gonna be okay," I said, my voice cracking with emotion. "Everything is gonna be okay." We cried in each other's arms, neither one of us wanting to let go first. But I finally pulled away to look at her. She looked years older than the Callie I had thought about earlier. It didn't matter. I was consumed with the idea that we were once again a family.

"Hey, Mom," Ann interrupted. "Let's show her some of your tricks."

I took a second to compose myself and soak in that look of pure joy on Callie's face. I watched her cry with delight as I walked the three steps to my bed by myself. She couldn't have been more elated.

In just a few minutes, Brint appeared at the door. I could see him through the window. He looked like he'd been crying. I motioned for him to come in.

He couldn't hide his tears after he entered the room. He grabbed me and gave me the biggest bear hug I think I've ever had.

"I thought you got worse," he said, not wanting to let go. "You're doing better?"

"You already missed her trick," Callie said quickly. "She can walk!"

I sat and looked at my three children before me. Complete happiness! Jubilation! I felt a bliss I never thought possible. All the horrific things that ravaged my being in the last month melted away. I was back. Therefore, my family was too.

Although my three babies were excited, they all looked exhausted and worried and unnerved. I was hesitantly anxious to hear their stories . . . *my* stories. . . what my life did to change theirs. But for the moment, I was languishing in just seeing them all together and happy.

"You made it," Ann said, proud of my accomplishment. "You really made it through this."

"No, Sweetie, *we* made it. I don't know what you all have been through, but I know I couldn't have gotten through it without you."

My kids beamed silently at our good turn of fortune. I took a mental photograph of the image before me. I never wanted to forget this moment for as long as I lived. I had a zillion questions, lots of work ahead of me, and an uncertain future, but it all kept coming back to one thing . . . my family really had made it through this crisis—together. Without their care and fortitude, I know I wouldn't have gotten better.

Dr. Hughes's prediction of my recovery astounded everyone. After weeks of researching and consulting, he concluded that I had been infected with Lyme disease, most likely from a tick. The first symptom of my illness probably was the grand mal seizure I had eight years ago. My disease grew more debilitating through the years, thus the other symptoms that crept up upon me like memory loss, balance issues and thought processing. There was less known about Lyme disease all those years ago, but it was now becoming more prevalent in Pennsylvania. It would not have been on a doctor's short list of diagnosis to choose from in 2004. Only within the past few years were people noticing the far-reaching and devastating effects this disease can produce.

Unfortunately, it had been difficult to diagnose my Lyme disease due to my reaction to Depakote. The seizures in early June from Lyme were most likely exacerbated by the drug. My severe memory issues, brain fog, and balance problems were all entwined with my drug reaction. Once the two troubles were separated, it was easier to see the differences between the two. Depakote was behind my dementia, my "going crazy" as my kids called it. It also caused brain damage. I still marvel at the reversibility of most of this damage. For so much harm to be done, then quickly erased, was something my family thought they'd never see.

Also, to my dismay, but probably to my advantage, I found that despite a rapid improvement in my memory recall, I couldn't remember anything from late May until August 3. Nothing from the rehab seemed familiar. I had no déjà vu. In fact, I could only remember snippets of the entire last three years and even those were cloudy.

During the recovery period that followed, it was hard for me to see my deficiencies. I told everyone I would be going back to work on August 25. I argued with those who thought it best to wait a bit. I talked to people as if I had just gotten over a cold instead of major trauma.

Since I had no memory of those months of craziness this summer, I was treating my life like it was the end of May. However, I was, in reality, far from normal. I needed speech therapy to retrain my mind, or trigger what I knew from before. It seemed silly to be asked such questions as, "Is a snowflake colder or hotter than a piece of toast?" and, "Can you name four ingredients used to make a cake?" And yet, I struggled with questions like these in the first few weeks. And no matter what my answers were, they were markedly better than the answers I had given all summer to "What is your name?" "Who is the president of the United States?" "Who is in your family?" These are all questions I had answered incorrectly just days before.

I also needed to learn to walk again. I was so proud of myself at the rehab when I actually took several steps without holding onto the railing. It was a very big deal!

When I was awarded my first day-pass to go home one Tuesday morning, I could not get over how much taller the trees were than I remembered. I didn't recall the bird feeder in the yard which we'd had for more than a year. I thought my family had changed the items around in the kitchen cupboards. I couldn't recall where anything was. I felt out of place in my own home! When it was time to go back to the rehab at the end of the day, I was relieved. Being a "visitor" at home brought me to tears at times. I just wanted everything to be back to the way it always was. I was given many more day-passes to visit home since therapy was still greatly needed to get me back to normal. The hours away from the rehab were welcome, but I still got tired and required care. I couldn't walk more than a few steps without assistance and my hands still trembled enough to make even me realize I wasn't ready to hold a glass of water.

After I was discharged on August 11, Home Nursing came daily to check my vitals and refill my pic line with antibiotics fighting the Lyme. Therapists came to my house to help me practice walking and strengthen my muscle tone. I was given exercises for my arms and legs and to relieve the pressure in my neck.

Language therapy was continued to develop my abilities to converse and translate thoughts into words. I still struggled with word-finding issues and needed to practice proper gender distinction. (I called my male cats: "she," and couldn't decipher the difference between "him" and "her" in a sentence.)

My small motor skills were challenged every time I tried to write, put on clothes, or eat. For months, I couldn't even hold a pencil. Now I was expecting myself to write sentences. My trembling hands struggled to write my name each day. In about a week, I was once again able to hold a beverage in my hand and use a straw to sip it. I would graduate to hot liquids but it would take many more weeks of practice. My tremors continued, however, Dr. Hughes felt with certainty they would go away. I had a lot of challenges in those first few months.

## 7 YEARS LATER

I make myself a cup of peppermint tea and head for the front porch. My iPad in hand, I am determined to spend the morning updating myself on the statistics of Lyme Disease. One would think, after such a harrowing experience, I would keep myself abreast of new treatments and progress made in the field of Lyme over the last several years. Instead, I've done the opposite. I've tried to ignore the disease, perhaps even deny I ever had Lyme. I've shied away from the advocates preaching tick recognition and safety. I've ignored articles on the later stages of Lyme. Aside from family and close friends, I never discuss my experience.

Well, it's been 7 years since that seizure I had in front of my students. I've had plenty of time to digest my malady and do some soul searching. But facing this all, head on, with the intention of teaching about it, was something I just couldn't bring myself to do. Until now.

I open up my iPad and type in Lyme Disease. Hundreds of sites come up. I scan the headings of each listing, searching for a medical center or other reputable source. I click on the first one I find.

I read down over the initial information. Symptoms and treatments are explained away in a smattering of a few sentences. I choose another site. This one lists a few more symptoms ignored in the last. My third choice, dwells on the phases of the disease. The next one discusses Lyme's effect on the skin. The amount of differing information is overwhelming! Listed treatments range anywhere from antibiotics to herbs to oils to prayer. I can't believe the diversity of the illness and its treatments!

For the first time in many years, I am scared. Up until now, I thought I had experienced the wrath of Lyme, gotten over it, and survived. Now I'm learning there are diseases one can get from the initial case of Lyme. Why hadn't anyone warned me of this? There are symptoms I currently have that I've dismissed, not realizing they can be byproducts of this horrendous disease. And then I read something that chills me to the bone—Lyme Disease does not go away! It becomes inactive! It can easily become active again at any time. One does not need another tick bite. I'm now petrified. My ignorance, my ridiculously strange aversion to researching progress in this disease is putting me at risk!

I take a sip of my tea and close my eyes. My heart is pounding. What if my Lyme is active again? What if my kids have Lyme and I don't know the latest warning signs? What if I am blocking out something about this infectious disease that I could use to prevent it?

I know Lyme is spreading, but I didn't realize its intensity or far reaching effects. I pull up Lyme on my screen again, wanting to get the most recent of statistics. I am mortified at what I find. Dates of informative articles range from the 1990's to 2018. I have to dig to even find a current article! And the most recent info for 2019 lists Lyme as the fastest growing vector-borne infectious disease in the US. The CDC (Center for Disease Control) says the latest estimate confirms Lyme infects more than 300,000 people a year. My mind reels as I find other facts:

1. The number of cases reported annually from the year 1997 to 2017 has had an increase of nearly 17,000 confirmed diagnoses (CDC, 2018.)
2. Though some individuals notice a tick bite right away, nearly half of others don't realize they have Lyme Disease until days or months after the infectious bite. .
3. The CDC currently advises a two-step testing process for Lyme Disease. If the first test result is found to be negative, no further testing is advised. This test often results in a false negative and some studies indicate this happens nearly 50 percent of the time.
4. There is no test available to prove that Lyme Disease is cured or the infectious bacteria is eradicated.
5. The bacterium Borrelia burgdorferi, which causes Lyme Disease, can trigger an auto-immune response causing symptoms that linger on well past the initial infection. This bacterium can also linger in an individual's system resulting in Post-Treatment Lyme Disease Syndrome (PTLDS.)
6. PTLDS has no treatment and although some doctors recommend a prolonged antibiotic, there is no proof at this time that patient's condition has improved.
7. The onset of Lyme Disease symptoms that the CDC provides, can be easily mistaken for other illness such as Alzheimer's, Multiple Sclerosis, Chronic Fatigue Syndrome, and others (CDC, 2019.) This occurs when symptoms for those illnesses are more evident or when another disease has already entered the central nervous system. This happens frequently when doctors are uninformed about Lyme Disease and do not test for borrelia burgdorferi.

I stand up and walk to the end of the porch. I look out over the yard and the splendor of the grass and trees. I am one of the lucky ones. I had an open-minded doctor who recognized, and treated the disease. Too many others may not have this luxury.

I feel the pangs of guilt. It wouldn't be right to keep my story secret. I need to help spread the word! I go back to my iPad and investigate support groups. Great! There is a local chapter that meets once a month. There are both state and national groups as well. There are chats with others who have Lyme and an abundance of fundraisers listed to aid in research.

I walk back to the kitchen for another cup of tea. My head is still swirling with the information I'd read. My desire to learn more is increasing by the minute.

My next mission is to find a list of ways to prevent Lyme disease. I sip my beverage while I scan the sites again, staying focused on sources with reputable backgrounds. When I come across the CDC's prevention strategies, I am excited to find there are ways to protect oneself from the horrors this disease can cause and to add additional strategies for keeping yourself tick free.

## HOW TO PROTECT YOURSELF AGAINST LYME DISEASE

1. Walk in the middle of trails and avoid leaning on trees (CDC, 2018.)
2. Use Environmental Protection Agency (EPA) insect repellant containing DEET.
3. Wear a hat to keep ticks off your scalp.
4. Wear a long-sleeved shirt that is fitted at your wrist.
5. Wear shoes and socks that cover your entire foot.
6. Consider permethrin for clothes.
7. Wear white or light-colored clothing to make it easier to see ticks.
8. Do tick checks immediately after coming indoors, especially in areas that sweat easily such as behind the knee caps and groin area.
9. Check for ticks again three days after outdoor activities.
10. If you find a tick, remove it carefully and save it for testing.
11. Treat your animals with tick repellant monthly to ensure they are not bringing them inside.

There are plenty more sites with additional ways to prevent Lyme. I scan through them, still shocked at how much information, and possibly misinformation, there is on the disease. My next job—finding the true symptoms of Lyme!

I know my own symptoms well. But learning about the full realm of problems is eye-opening! The various symptoms that can occur when someone is bitten by an infectious tick is truly endless.

I close my iPad and stretch. I am having a mixture of feelings from disbelief to anxiety to denial. There is no way for me to describe the spectrum of chaos and danger this disease is capable of. After my hours of research, I feel like yelling from the roof tops to warn everyone. I certainly wish I had known about it earlier. That initial seizure I had in Lowe's fourteen years ago was most likely the beginning for me. And yet, my chances of realizing I had this disease at that time were minimal. I'd never even heard of the condition until six years later.

There is so much to learn! My initial task is sorting out the reputable sites and pouring over the information. It's a long process, and one I wish I had started a long time ago. I now realize my illness has reached Stage 3. Some of the symptoms I read about are present in me. I still have major memory problems. In fact, I've lost at least three years of memories that I'll never get back. I've developed Celiac's Disease as a byproduct of Lyme. I've gone through menopause twice, due to Lyme Disease, and have hormones that skyrocket from one end to the other in a moment's notice. I still tire easily and the fogginess in my brain has taken up residency there.

I make myself a toasted cheese sandwich and open a can of tomato soup. I wonder, how many professionals, from pharmacists to doctors to nurses, look over prescriptions and neglect to associate side effects with symptoms? How much harm have the side effects already done to my body? Are there other people out there, in nursing homes or other health facilities, where a prescription is responsible for their issues? If Dr. Hughes had not identified the source of my dementia, where would I be now?

So many worries! But that will be for another day. I survived. And I survived for a reason. God saw me through my daily struggles. He gave me and my family the strength to trudge through the darkness when we were all feeling hopeless. Now, I am finally ready to fully diagram the scope of my crisis. I am strong enough now to turn my misfortune into a gain for others.

I do realize Lyme will always be with me. But, so will God. He's paved my pathway to use this tumultuous turmoil for the better. It has been a daunting journey already, but I trust him to see me through to the end.

Life can be trying and difficult, just as it can be wonderful and fascinating. We must accept our days here on earth gratefully, and live them for others as well as ourselves. Cherish friendships and forgive unkind acts. And always remember family. You will be rewarded in the end. As Hunter and I often remind each other now, "God is good."

www.ingramcontent.com/pod-product-compliance
Lightning Source LLC
Chambersburg PA
CBHW062002180426
43198CB00036B/2147